Self
Development

Learn the Healing Powers of Reiki to Awaken
Your Chakras & Achieve Piece of Mind

(Increase Positive Energy, Boost Vitality, and
Improve Health)

Llyn Bevell

Published by Rob Miles

Llyn Bevell

All Rights Reserved

Self Development: Learn the Healing Powers of Reiki to Awaken Your Chakras & Achieve Piece of Mind (Increase Positive Energy, Boost Vitality, and Improve Health)

ISBN 978-1-989990-36-0

All rights reserved. No part of this guide may be reproduced in any form without permission in writing from the publisher except in the case of brief quotations embodied in critical articles or reviews.

Legal & Disclaimer

The information contained in this book is not designed to replace or take the place of any form of medicine or professional medical advice. The information in this book has been provided for educational and entertainment purposes only.

The information contained in this book has been compiled from sources deemed reliable, and it is accurate to the best of the Author's knowledge; however, the Author cannot guarantee its accuracy and validity and cannot be held liable for any errors or omissions. Changes are periodically made to this book. You must consult your doctor or get professional medical advice before using any of the suggested remedies, techniques, or information in this book.

Upon using the information contained in this book, you agree to hold harmless the Author from and against any damages, costs, and expenses, including any legal fees potentially resulting from the application of any of the information provided by this guide. This disclaimer applies to any damages or injury caused by the use and application, whether directly or indirectly, of any advice or information presented, whether for breach of contract, tort, negligence, personal injury, criminal intent, or under any other cause of action.

You agree to accept all risks of using the information presented inside this book. You need to consult a professional medical practitioner in order to ensure you are both able and healthy enough to participate in this program.

TABLE OF CONTENTS

INTRODUCTION 1

CHAPTER 1: GETTING STARTED: YOUR ULTIMATE GUIDE TO REIKI 3

CHAPTER 2: BENEFITS OF REIKI 17

CHAPTER 3: THE POWER AND BENEFITS OF ENERGY HEALING 25

CHAPTER 4: TYPES OF REIKI HEALING 34

CHAPTER 5: AN ENERGY BY ANY OTHER NAME IS STILL THE SAME 53

CHAPTER 6: ESTABLISHING YOUR INTENT 64

CHAPTER 7: THE HUMAN ENERGY BODY 70

CHAPTER 8: GETTING STARTED 80

CHAPTER 9: THE HISTORY OF REIKI 89

CHAPTER 10: THE REIKI LEVELS AND ATTUNEMENTS 106

CHAPTER 11: AN INTRODUCTION TO REIKI 118

CHAPTER 12: THE PLANES OF EXISTENCE 122

CHAPTER 13: THE REIKI DIVISION 142

CHAPTER 14: OTHER SELF-HEALING TECHNIQUES 151

CHAPTER 15: UNDERSTANDING THE REIKI SYMBOLS 169

CHAPTER 16: TESTIMONIALS AND STORIES 174

CHAPTER 17: MENTAL, EMOTIONAL, AND SPIRITUAL HEALING 190

CONCLUSION 206

Introduction

Illness and maladies are a perpetual part of our life, and always have been – slowly the demand for effective, holistic and natural forms of treatment has risen because people are losing their faith in artificial forms of chemical medication. This is why the Reiki system of natural healing through spiritual energy has taken the world by storm, and people want to know how this miraculous system works. The popularity of Reiki has risen because of its proven benefits, and its ability to heal not just the physical, but also the mind, and the spirit.

Reiki works through the abundant universal life force energy that flows through the whole cosmos. Reiki is based on the mystical logic of life, which assumes that the reason why we get ill is that the energy in our body is imbalanced or some negative energy has seeped into the body. The purpose of Reiki is not just to make you aware of this flow of energy inside you but also to teach you how to harness this energy and heal through it. To make it simpler, you can understand this energy as the concept of 'light' in Christianity or 'Chi' in traditional Chinese culture.

Reiki has numerous benefits, but its primary purpose is to restore the energy you have lost or to disperse the negative energy you have accumulated. The loss of vitality in the modern world is what makes it difficult for us to get up in the morning – Reiki restores this vitality, by rejuvenating your spirit, body and mind.

In this book, we will start by first understanding what Reiki means, its traditional definitions and philosophical basis, and its vibrant and deep history. Next is a look into the principles on which Reiki is based, the various ways to practice Reiki on yourself and others, and the use of symbols in Reiki. In the last part of the book, we will have an in-depth discussion on the basics of Reiki learning, how you can become a Reiki master, and start your practice.

Chapter 1: Getting Started: Your Ultimate Guide To Reiki

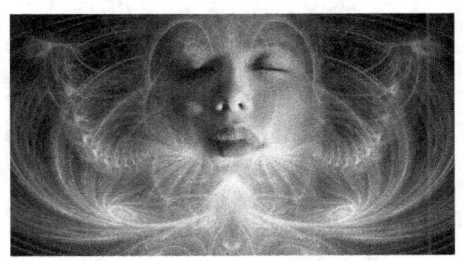

What is Reiki?

Reiki is a gentle form of therapy that involves touch and is meant to assist the body to heal itself from common ailments that it is dealing with. Reiki practitioners are able to tap into the natural energy of the body in order to remove any blockage that may be there and to redirect the flow of misdirected or stagnant energy that is there. This can help to promote the health and wellness inside the individual.

Reiki is going to rely on helping the chakras, or the energy centers, of the body. These energy centers are going to allow the practitioner to stimulate the healing abilities that are found naturally inside of the body. Through straightening, healing, and clearing the flow of energy through the body, it is possible to resolve many of the common ailments that are going on inside of the body, including emotional, mental, and physical problems.

When you do not take care of your energy imbalances, it is going to cause some physical ailments inside of the body. In fact, many of the diseases and illnesses that go on inside the body are due to these energy imbalances. Reiki is able to come in and solve some of these problems, opening up those energy centers so that you feel much better. Reiki is also known as a form of mental therapy because it has the ability to impact your psychological conditions, like depression and anxiety, in a positive manner. In fact, those who have practiced Reiki often feel a better sense of well-being and improved self-confidence when they are done.

Reiki can work well for so many people because it is gentle and non-invasive, which is completely different compared to the other forms of alternative healing Rather than focusing all that energy on the symptoms of a condition, Reiki is going to treat the whole person, helping to send healing energy in the direction that it is needed the most.

Preparation Before Your Session

To first prepare your mind, you'll want to speak the Reiki Ideals. Say the words from your heart and mind, as well as your lips.

As you are repeating the Reiki Ideas, put your hands, palms together, in front of your heart chakra as illustrated on the following pages. Before you begin, invite your inner spirit to participate in this self-healing process. You will be the healer and the healed as you practice Reiki's self-healing discipline.

Think of this as a Reiki prayer. It should be done with a reverent and open heart. This is not a time to be skeptical or doubtful, but rather a time of knowing that you are about to be introduced to your helper and comforter, your strength and guide. Breathe deeply; focus on slowly inhaling through your nose and then just as slowly exhaling through your mouth. When you have released all the air from your lungs, let your breath drift off then hold it for about five to six seconds longer before slowly releasing the remaining air from your passageways.

Invite Reiki to guide your energy throughout every cell of your body, touching the areas that require healing. Continue to feel the relaxing rhythm of your heart as Reiki responds to your gentle requests for calmness, peace, and healing.

To be completely prepared for your session, do this first Reiki pose each evening for three or four days before your full session to come. This will help to open your chakras and encourage your mind to freely and fearlessly seek Reiki before your first session and be fully prepared to release what binds you.

Only ask and invite during these first few evenings, staying calm and relaxed, prayerfully seeking Reiki's wisdom and healing power for your first full session. Remember to thank Reiki for all that you are about to experience. Make sure you get plenty of rest and drink lots of water to wash away the negatives.

Symbols: Reiki has its own three sets of symbols representing its own arena or its own category of assumptions. The first is Tattwa. Tattwa has five different symbols each representing a different element of the universe. They represent earth, air, water, fire, spirit. They reign over the realm of energy in the brain. This group of symbols may also affect other areas such as realities that are not physical like dreams.

The next symbol group is physical items such as Rosaries. They have the ability to be charged with the power to cause an effect. The final group of devices like the Reiki symbols learned earlier, that can enable the use of Reiki energy. These symbols offer a pathway to connection with energy that is independent.

The symbols are not the exclusive means of accessing Reiki energy. They will make your Reiki experience much more gratifying or satisfying. If you don't know the exact meaning of any given symbol you may still use it; you will gain wisdom with time and practice.

The Master Symbol of Reiki holds the greatest power. It is used for a much deeper, spiritual healing. It enhances one's intuition and can change your life dramatically. The Master Reiki symbol is made of three kanji's (characters). One means great or greatly. The second means light in noun form or smooth as an adjective. This kanji may also mean completely. The final kanji is an adjective or a verb. It may mean evident or see, understand. Put together, the three kanji's mean great bright light.

Remember, you may use all or only selected symbols, they are not a necessary ingredient in Reiki. They do bring enhancement to the energy flow. You may, of course, choose to use none.

Like earlier mentioned symbols, these can be activated in numerous ways. You might draw or visualize a symbol, or you may chant. You might form the shape in your mouth with the tip of your tongue. How you activate is up to you.

Prepare your chakras: Prior to using Reiki meditation on yourself, you are going to want to ensure that your chakras are open and ready for the experience as well. The following technique will also work well with the Kundalini meditation discussed in the next chapter. While you are welcome to work through the entire process each time, you may instead simply want to focus on the parts that deal with the chakras that are bothering you the most.

For starters, you will work on the root chakra which you can start doing by simply focusing on the color red. When you start focusing on the color the odds are pretty good that it is a dull, dark red as opposed to a strong, vibrant red which should be your ultimate goal. Throughout your time working with this chakra you are going to want to focus on the color until it is bright and pulsating.

After you have opened up your root chakra, you will be ready to move on to the sacral chakra which is associated with the color orange which you will want to focus on making shine as brightly as possible. In fact, each chakra has its own color and you will want to focus on it as you work to make that particular chakra shine. You will want to make your way up the body until you reach the crown chakra. Once you have done so you can expect all of your chakras to be fully opened which means you are ready to move forward with Reiki meditation.

It is important to understand that this method is not something that you are going to see results with overnight. Depending on how tarnished your chakras are it could take weeks of diligent effort to get them shining brightly. Thus, if this is your first time with this practice or you simply haven't done it in a while then it is important to leave yourself enough time to do it properly without feeling rushed.

Gassho meditation: Another technique that you are able to use is known as Gassho Meditation. This method is going to take about five to fifteen minutes where you will focus all of your attention just on Reiki. It is beneficial to do this for each day, although there are programs that will help you to get started and they recommend doing it for 21-days to see how you like it.

The steps to Gassho meditation are pretty simple. You do not need to do a ton of things other than concentrate on the Reiki healing powers, do some deep breathing, and sit in the right position. The steps that you need for Gassho Meditation include:

- Take your hands and hold them in a prayer position. This is traditionally leaving the hands, with palms together, touching and the fingers touching as well. Make sure that these prayer hands are right at the heart.
- When the hands are done, close your eyes.
- Start to breathe in the Reiki energy through your nose, taking in a nice deep breath rather than the fast and uneven breaths that you have been doing before.
- Once you are ready, it is time to exhale that breath through your whole body. This would include the physical body, the

etheric body, the mental body, and the spiritual body.

You would just keep on with the deep breathing for as long as you needed, concentrating on the Reiki healing power as you go. Of course, there are a few different variations that you can try with this. Some people like to add these in because they allow them something to concentrate on or because they think that it adds some more power.

You can choose to write down a goal and then ask that some sort of clarification comes to you throughout your session. You can add in some music, as long as it is soft and inspiring in some manner or even chants a mantra. If you are dealing with a big problem in your life, you could ask for some help and guidance to get through that problem. And some people decide to draw the power symbol, the mental or emotional symbol, or the distance symbol over their body when they first get started. You are able to choose the variation that works the best for you, or you can stick with the steps that are listed above to help you.

Reiki Meditation Example

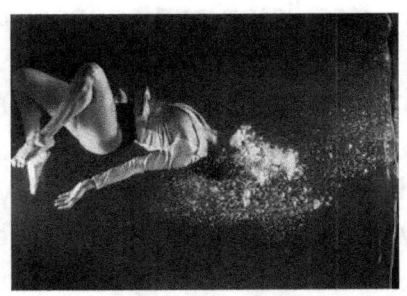

Lay or sit down comfortably on a mat. Keep your back straight. Stay relaxed, composed, and calm. Breathe deeply. Imagine that you are inhaling the goodness and happiness that you want. Now exhale all the negative emotions like anxiety, fear, and depression. Imagine them leaving your body. Do this a few times and think about how in tune your mind and body are. Just relax.

There are seven different chakras in the body. They go from the bottom of your spine to the top of your head. These are energy centers for the body. Put your hand in front of each chakra and hold it for a few minutes. This all depends on what your body needs. If your body asks for it to stay longer, leave it there. Move it if the body has enough. Feeling with the hands is the best way to listen and connect to your body. As you tune in with your hands, imagine the universe's life force is entering your body through the hands.

Your chakras are the passageway. Feel your body vibrate with the energy flow. Go into deep relaxation and rejuvenation.

Put your palms together at the top of your head. Hold your hands there and listen to your body. Pay attention. Continue to do this and breathe slowly and deeply. Remove all the negative and bring all the positives into you. Relax.

Put your hands on your forehead. Now move them to the back of your head. Move down to the throat and put on hand on the throat and the other at the back of the neck. Hold this for a time and relax.

Continue down and put your hands on the back of your shoulders. Your fingers should be facing downward. Your touch needs to be gentle. Hold your hands still until the body is ready for it to be moved.

Put your hands on your chest covering your heart. Remember to hold until the body tells you to move.

Move on to the rib area, then the stomach and lower abdomen. Keeping your touch gentle and moving when the body is ready.

When you are done with the head and torso, move to the hips and put your hands on both your hips. Moving only when the body tells you to. Feel the energy flowing through the body. Enjoy the sensations.

Move on to your knees and feet. For your feet, place the hands either on bottom or top whichever is more comfortable. Move your hands when your body is ready. Enjoy the experience.

Finally, place your hands in the prayer position and put them in front of your chest. Sit with the spine straight and the body taut. Breathe normally. Feel the energy coursing through your body. Continue this for another three to five minutes or as long as you feel the need. This process is done when you feel energized and ignited.

Chapter 2: Benefits Of Reiki

One of the biggest questions you may have is, "Why Reiki?" There are dozens, possibly even hundreds, of forms of meditation, yoga and other holistic healing practices designed to promote this overall feeling of wellness and stave off sickness and negative emotions. Even though there are many options, Reiki sets itself apart because of how easy it is — you can do it anywhere, without any equipment, at any time of the day. Aside from the convenience factor, this chapter will go over some of the benefits of regular Reiki practice.

Helps with Physical Healing

Physical healing is one of the benefits of Reiki that people seem to be most skeptical about. They do not understand how something that restores energy can help relieve the symptoms of their physical condition, whether it is a dull headache or a chronic illness. Those who doubt this method have often been healed using a Western form of medicine, which commonly focuses on treating the ailment directly instead of using a full-body approach. This is one of the reasons that people turn to alternative or holistic medicine when a more scientific approach has healed them. In many cases, the results have been a complete turnaround. There are even anecdotes of people who have turned to Reiki healing and other alternative medicines and had success in healing cancer, relieving chronic pain, and fighting off severe illness.

Helps with Spiritual Healing

The flow of energy that you experience with Reiki can help you notice the interconnectedness between all the life forms of earth. As you connect to all that is living around you, you will feel a greater connection to the divine. You will also feel as if you are part of something higher than what exists in your immediate world. For many people, this creates the feeling of being connected to something great and powerful. It offers reassurance that you are present in the Universe and you know that you are loved by and connected to the spiritual beings, both living and non-living that you may encounter through your day.

Helps with Mental and Emotional Healing

People's pain and sickness are not always visible. Many people struggle with anxiety, depression, repressed emotions, and other mental and emotional states. They may not even be aware of their emotional state or what is causing it. Reiki does not always help you heal emotions unless you deal with them. However, it can make you more aware of your emotional state. This awareness can help you understand your problems. It can also help you tap into the divine nature and understand your purpose in life. As you continue to connect to the energy that exists within everything and all around you, it can help cultivate more positive emotions in your life, including connectedness, love, intimacy, kindness, compassion, and sharing.

Helps to Deal with Stress and Negative Energy Created by the World

We cannot always control whom we interact with. Even in the best careers, we might have to work with people that give off generally bad energies or who take advantage of others. You may pick up negativity from encountering an angry person at the bus stop or the coffee shop. You might even have your own negative emotions to deal with, as feeling sad or angry at times is part of the human experience.

The benefit of Reiki is that it helps relieve you of the weight of any negative experiences you may have. As you walk through your office building or down the street, you will notice a new recognition for those things that do not serve your purpose. You will understand what things do not serve your purpose in life and which encounters leave you in an undesirable mental state. Then, you can learn to block the energies from things you do not want to experience and avoid those situations that you can, should they not promote the happy, energized feeling that you should feel.

Increases Compassion for Others

The connectedness that you feel when regularly cleansing and connecting to your internal source of energy can help you find greater compassion for all that exists in the world. You will be more compassionate and empathetic when you encounter others who are in pain, whether emotional or physical. You will also be more tolerant and understanding of others, aware that you cannot possibly understand their specific situation. As you learn this deep compassion for others, you will also learn to be kinder to and have greater compassion for yourself. This can help heal people who struggle with emotional trauma or low self-esteem, as they often struggle with treating themselves as well as they would treat others.

Helps to Heal Others

If you decide to progress past the point of Reiki healing for yourself, it is easy to become attuned with the world and direct your energy in a way that corrects the energy flow of others. As you choose people to practice with, it is essential to choose those that are open to the idea of Reiki healing. You may find yourself put off by the practice altogether if you try it on a relative with health problems who do not have an open mind to new age topics like Reiki. Keep in mind that it is not always your failure. Reiki will not work on someone who cannot open his or her mind and body to the flow of energy.

Stress Relief

Stress relief is a significant benefit of Reiki, as it is responsible for many of its effects. When you regularly relax and provide yourself with stress relief, it gives your body and minds a much-needed break from the fast-paced world around you. This stress relief can help you sleep better at night and promotes a stronger immune system since your body is getting the support that it needs to be healthy. This can also reduce blood pressure.

Body and Mind Detoxification

A significant part of the Reiki process is the removal of negative energies and toxins from your body. It cleanses the body and helps you naturally eliminate toxins that may have built up in your organs, digestive system, and bloodstream. You naturally encounter these toxins through your day— they are in some of the foods that you eat and the air that you breathe. Reiki also detoxifies the mind, clearing it of blockages that are stopping you from dealing with emotional trauma. This more lucid state of mind and deeper understanding help you on the path to healing.

Energizing and Rejuvenating

Reiki is a very energizing practice. As you tap into your own spiritual energy and the connectedness between you and all that is in the Universe, you will feel your energy grow. You will feel reinvigorated as the life force flows through your body. Some Reiki experts also say that the rejuvenation from Reiki can postpone the aging process and promote overall vitality.

Reiki is something that can take several attempts to get right. By knowing the benefits, you can be sure you are committing to a healing process. Reiki is worth learning, whether you use it to improve the quality of your own life or to transfer your energy to heal someone else.

Chapter 3: The Power And Benefits Of Energy Healing

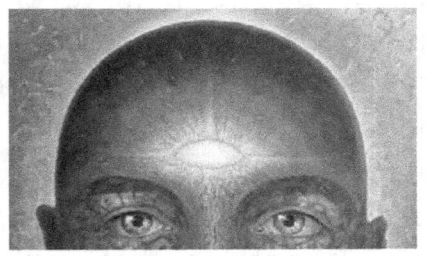

Consider the idea of electricity for a moment. We have found ways to harness energy in which it can be created almost instantaneously, travel miles and miles to your home to power all of our daily appliances, all in a matter of milliseconds. In the worst cases, lightning can strike from a thunder cloud a mile into the atmosphere and incinerate its target before it even knew what happened. Electricity is so powerful that it can be dangerous if not used carefully.

Luckily for us, humans hover at a much lower energy frequency, hardly even close to the capacity of pure energy. However, some people can harness and use more energy than others. Maybe you have noticed that a friend or co-worker is always energized and ready to go. Perhaps they are simply pulling in more energy from the universe than you, and have it to burn. You can learn to harness this energy by fixing your energy flow and tapping into your full potential.

Since the entire universe is made up of energy, there is nothing that can't be improved via energy healing. With proper care, your body can work to its fullest potential without ailment and disease. Your emotional state can improve, with less stress and more happiness overall. You can attract people that value you and bring joy to your life. You can be successful professionally and personally beyond your wildest dreams if you simply tap into the energy that is already inside of you.

In order to get these results, we must know where you are starting from. Imagine your body as multiple strings of Christmas lights. Even if you do not celebrate, you are likely well aware of the pitfalls of these brightly colored strings of light. Hundreds of tiny bulbs are strung together by tiny, fragile wires. Every string can be connected to another, to eventually light up the tree, the house, or whatever else needs some cheer.

As the fragile wires and bulbs age, they become brittle and are more likely to lose electrical connection and fail. The dimming of one bulb may not have an effect on the aesthetics of your Christmas tree, but that's also not how it works. The problem is, each of those light bulbs is connected and requires the light before it to work for them all to work. So, if one goes out, they all go out. The energy cannot flow properly, and the holiday festivities come to a sudden halt.

The energy in your body works the same way. Our bodies are made up of systems of nerves that flow through every tissue, every organ. If one connection is lost, the whole system of energy is thrown off, and the body cannot work properly. One of the most obvious physiological examples of this is carpal tunnel syndrome. This is usually caused by a pinched nerve under the shoulder blade that prevents the entire arm from working properly. Sufferers experience pain and tingling and can be debilitating. Many cases can be resolved with physical therapy that removes pressure off of the affected nerve to restore energy balance to the arm.

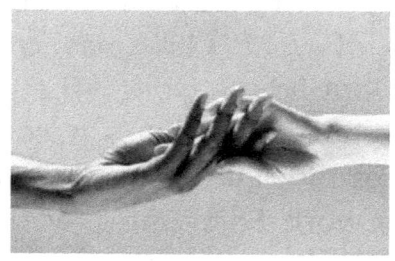

Most energy healing is done through light touch between one person and another. Usually, a trained professional, the healer, is at the center of the work, and the patient is on the receiving end of the energy. As energy is of a fluent nature, it is possible to transfer energy from one person to another, and this is the basis of the healing properties.

This transfer of energy is done in a quiet, relaxed environment, like when getting a massage. Most people who partake in this healing feel a deep sense of relaxation during and after the treatment. Reducing this stress brings about a great change in the body, as muscles and nerves relax, getting back to their normal, functional state.

Specific energy healing is done to focus on the endocrine glands as well. This system is responsible for releasing toxins from the body, and if energy is blocked around this area, the toxic matter is allowed to build up in the body, causing lethargy, illness, and disease. Moving energy to this area promotes proper function and flushes toxins properly from the body. As these toxins are removed naturally, the immune system improves as well. If this system was formerly trying to eliminate these toxins, making the body more susceptible to attack, illness is much more likely. Removing this burden from the immune system increases overall wellness.

Energy healing can also help with small ailments as it boosts the immune system. Head colds, arthritis, general pain and inflammation can all disappear when properly and frequently treated with energy healing. Fixing energy pathways can reduce headaches, as energy and proper blood flow is restored to the brain.

The power of energy healing is also an important tool in chronic and serious illness, like cancer treatment. Generally, traditional treatments like chemotherapy and radiation are very taxing procedures that actually harm the body. Heavy chemicals and radiation are meant to kill off the cancer cells, but end up harming healthy cells as well. The body loads more energy to restore the healthy cells and often leads to symptoms of fatigue, malaise muscle loss and much more. The body requires a higher intake of energy from food to maintain this rebuilding process, but often symptoms of nausea and decreased appetite from treatment prevent this from happening.

Energy healing can help transfer energy from the universe into that body to help out. Also, unblocking energy channels can help things flow more freely, making it easier for the body to recover. Energy healing, combined with a proper, nutrient-rich diet can help the body produce the energy it needs to fight and recover from the disease.

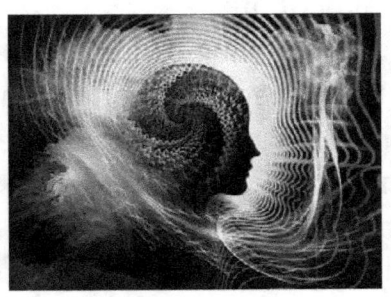

Perhaps the most important benefit of energy healing is restoring emotional balance. As we know, emotions are centered in the brain, and they are manifested as hormones are released in the brain. If hormone balance is off even the slightest bit, it can cause us to become moody, depressed and anxious, among a host of other problems. If you have ever experienced this, whether, for a short time or a long duration, you know how great of an impact it has on your overall health and life. Feeling depressed sucks your energy, makes you feel achy and generally sluggish. You can't concentrate on tasks, and socializing with others feels like a chore. Feeling this way for long periods of time can affect your social ties, career and overall quality of life.

Using energy healing to unblock energy channels that affect hormone balance is a great remedy to try. The feeling of relaxation and revitalization that accompanies an energy healing session may be all you need to get your hormones back in balance, and to start feeling well again.

The power of energy healing is actually boundless. Regularly partaking in energy healing sessions can improve health and emotional wellness across the board, leading to a better quality of life overall. Finding help from a practiced healer is your best bet, but it is possible to practice energy healing on yourself as well. More on that in the following chapters.

Chapter 4: Types Of Reiki Healing

There are two types of Reiki Healing: Hands-on and Distant.

Hands-on healing is where the palms of a healer are three to five inches from your body. There are certain points on a person's body that are called chakras. The healer will heal a person at those points on the body. When there are several people in a group having hands-on treatments, it becomes much more powerful.

Using a series of hand techniques, a skilled Reiki healer will infuse this life force energy into any disrupted fields to clear blockage and thereby restore normal function. By researching, studying, and strengthening your own awareness, in combination with Reiki symbols, these powerful principles can be used for self-healing and healing of others.

Distant healing can be performed at any time at any place. Patients don't have to be close to the healer and, indeed, those in need of healing have been known to receive it from practically the other side of the world. All a healer needs is some of your personal information like your name, age, and photograph. This healing process is as effective and powerful as the hands-on healing.

Reiki healing works to provide you with energy to cope with and fight the negativity both inside and outside of your body. Many people have given testimonials about how greatly they have benefited from Reiki healing. Some patients with major illnesses like cancer and AIDS have reportedly been cured using Reiki healing.

The duration of the healing will depend on the severity of the problem. If it is minor, such as a cold with fever or sinus issues, healing will take up to one week, but could take less. If the problem is more severe or chronic such as diabetes, or cancer, then healing could take several weeks or even months.

When a Reiki symbol is used by the practitioner, the symbol will then let the practitioner send their energy through space to where it can do the most good. It can also work with a person directly to clear and heal any blockages that might have formed, regardless of how long they may have existed in the subject. Geographic locations or even communities can also be cleansed all at once by these energy powers.

Over the years, many new Reiki styles have been developed, including other "distance" healing concepts. Then, the idea of applying Reiki to groups of people, places, and situations was developed. These newer Reiki healing principles differ from the original Usui Reiki method for body and mind.

So, if you are referring the original Reiki practice, the maximum number of people for whom one can perform a Reiki session remotely is two at a time, but one at a time is preferred.

To perform distant Reiki sessions, you first need to fill your hands with power using chakras and the Usui symbol of power. Then, apply the Reiki principles on yourself for about fifteen minutes, followed by visualizing the Reiki type that is for distance and that healing symbol while saying the name for a total of three repetitions. You will need to visualize the person you want to send your energy to as well.

It doesn't matter if you are in another part of the world, you can connect with anyone by using distant Reiki to gain direction and clarity in relationships, health, business, and personal issues.

Distant Reiki reconnects you to your inner being so you can accomplish anything with confidence.

Benefits of Distant Reiki are:
- Increases energy
- Decreases feelings of pain and stress
- Increases feelings of love and openness
- Increases ability to gladly take on new challenges
- Improves quality of sleep
- Improves interpersonal communication
- Faster recovery after surgeries or sickness
- Become more in tune with your

emotions
- Clears your mind
- Inspires creativity
- Improves weight loss
- Improves fertility
- Increases confidence
- Reduces grief
- Improves the immune system
- Eases sorrow
- Decreases the desire for addictive behavior

By creating your own self-healing path, you are helping yourself and others. Through your spiritual and personal growth, you will advance human consciousness using your own skills and learn to nurture and love yourself and others. You will be stronger, happier, and offer a better healing experience for other people as a result.

Here are some important points for Reiki and self-healing journeys:

In practicing Reiki healing, you must trust yourself and trust that you have the knowledge and the experience as a healer to connect to the divine power of healing and love. Give yourself the necessary time to heal yourself as you help and heal other people. You will feel confident and satisfied that you are able to give healing energy to not only yourself but to others as well.

Meditate every day by using whatever experience you have. The use of meditation to heal yourself is crucial to being able to heal others. Understanding yourself is a guide you will use to seek the divine presence to create the important union you must possess. Make it your goal to understand yourself in all ways to create a happier, more balanced, and healthy life for yourself.

Meditation has been a core part of countless different cultural beliefs since time immemorial. It is a proven way to help a person achieve inner tranquility and peace, exist more fully in the moment, and understand the true connection between the mind, soul, and body. Getting into the swing of it can sound difficult especially if you are unfamiliar with the basics. But the truth is, it is actually easy. The following practices are a great way to start getting in touch with your energy before taking on the responsibility of Reiki energy:

When you first awaken in the morning, before you even open your eyes and get out of bed, take a minute to listen to all the sounds that surround you as you start the day. While doing so, try to block out all of the thoughts that typically swarm into your mind at the start of the day and all the worries and responsibilities that you are going to need to deal with before you can crawl back into bed once more. Making a concentrated effort to silence those thoughts first thing will make it easier to maintain a clear mind throughout the day.

Another good way to get in the habit of regular meditation is to simply become more aware of the way you breathe on a regular basis. As you breathe in, consider just what it is you are doing, focus on taking long, deep, soothing breaths, in and out, in and out. With enough practice, you won't need to think about breathing correctly – it will become something you will just do naturally. What's more, being able to easily focus on it will help you to get your mind back on track if it ends up wandering in the future during other meditative exercises.

While breathing, you are going to want to ensure that you inhale with your diaphragm rather than your chest before letting the breath expand to your lungs. Doing so will help to ensure that you breathe in as deeply as your body is able. It will also help to slow your overall breathing which will reduce your heart rate, naturally reinforcing the idea that you are calming your body as well as your mind.

You are going to want to start with just this small mediation for a time before letting the amount of time you do so at once grow longer and longer. Start with a goal of remaining free from distraction for one minute, then five, ten and so on. The actual length that you practice for in a day isn't as important as the fact that you use the time to clear your mind and become more aware of the connection between your body and your mind.

When you are first starting out, try to meditate for at least five minutes per day, broken up into periods that you can remain fully focused on the moment for. Take some time in the morning to practice, and then again during the mid-afternoon as a counter to the after-lunch slump. Finally, end your day with another meditation session to ensure you are properly relaxed and ready for bed. If you keep at it, you should start to notice an improvement in both body and spirit in just a few weeks. You will likely find that you have more energy, are generally happier, and overall more relaxed.

What to Expect

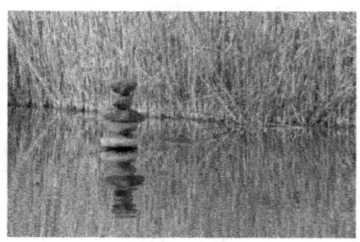

During a healing session, the practitioner will focus on "chakras" (energy points) and will use a very light touch or hold the patient's hands above the chakras to start the healing process and spiritual cleansing. The patient may feel some tingling or warming sensations during this healing process. Each person may experience different sensations, and some may not even feel anything.

Reiki involves positive experiences in your physical, emotional and spiritual health. When you leave a session, you will be amazed to discover how relaxed you are, to the point that you may even experience complete tranquility. With practice, you will be able to begin to do Reiki at home for yourself or your family after learning from a qualified healer.

You need to be attuned to Reiki in order to practice the technique on yourself. This can be accomplished by taking a Level-1 course with a Reiki Master.

If you are considering doing "self-Reiki," it is important that you attend a class because there are techniques that are only taught in a class. There you will learn where to tap the healing energy correctly.

It is also important to consider what type of Reiki you are naturally drawn to. There is the Usui Reiki western style, which is probably the most common. It would be very easy to find a teacher for this style. Online Reiki classes are not recommended because Reiki is a hands-on healing art. Reiki can be shared with others by passing on attunements that awaken the energy.

The steps of Reiki attunement are simple to learn but complicated to master.

You need to have a quiet place to comfortably sit or lie down. Use a small room or anywhere you will not be interrupted by people or noise. Then practice these steps while following your own breath:

Place your tongue's tip on the roof of your mouth and breathe in slowly through your nose. You will notice the air entering your nose and filling your lungs.

Next, lower your tongue and exhale slowly. Notice the path of your breath when it moves out of your lungs, into your throat and over your tongue.

Repeat these steps three times. If you have difficulty quieting your mind or have other distractions, just take a break. After a little bit just return to your space and begin again. To quiet your mind, just repeat to yourself, "I am inhaling, one… I am exhaling, two..." Or count your inhalation and exhalation, "1, 2, 3," etc.

Practice this breathing technique throughout your day. Think about your breath, concentrating on each inhalation and exhalation, stretch, and notice the sensations of the muscles and skin.

This will develop your sensitivity and help you to become more aware of your environment. This can sometimes be overwhelming. So do not hesitate to take breaks. No one can do this all day, but five minutes a day will be a great goal to start with.

During your sessions, you might notice distress, aches, pain, or even anger. Notice also where these feelings are coming from and listen to your body. When you locate the source of such feelings, you will want to focus all of your energy on removing any related blockages you might find. With practice, you will find that you can feel a physical heat over the blockage when you focus on it. Emotions want to be noticed. This exercise will teach you to develop your energy healing without Reiki.

Reiki Frequency Session Planning

As far as the frequency of Reiki attunements, in general, if you compare it with physical therapy, regular weekly sessions are better than randomly taking a session once in a while – just like visiting a gym once a month won't help you to lose weight. Also, it depends on the Reiki practitioner and their experience if they can go deeper in a single session.

Most clients notice an effect after one session although some need more sessions before they really notice a change in themselves. Fortunately, there is nothing you need to "do" or "prepare for" prior to a session. Just relax and enjoy the healing powers. A good schedule is:

- The first week, plan 3–4 sessions in

consecutive days. Then, take a break for a few days.
- The next week, plan 2–3 sessions.
- After that, plan one session per week.

Each session will last for one hour. Typically, most clients don't need to come back after eight sessions.

There are three levels of Reiki healing that can be reached through practice and education. A Reiki Master opens and expands energy channels to people who want to learn this spiritual energy force healing. Some, for their own well-being and others, to become a healing practitioner. Reiki attunement is performed to open and clear blockages to empower the highest abundance of energy to flow into a person's body and mind for the ultimate health and well-being. You must have a total commitment to Reiki to become a Reiki master.

The Reiki degree levels are explained here:

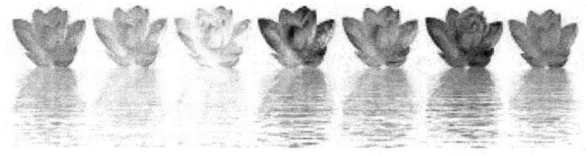

Reiki Level 1

Level 1 Reiki focuses on opening energy forces which gives the practitioner the ability to connect to the universal energy. This energy moves into the top of the person and flows into the mind, down to the heart and finally, moves through the hands.

The goal of level 1 is using self-Reiki, and masters encourage people who want to reach this level, to focus on practicing this energy healing on themselves. They will then learn to work through stumbling blocks they may come upon through practice and repetition. Many masters experience their own physical symptoms of energy in their hands when performing their first attunement, including cooling, heating, or tingling sensations.

Reiki Level 2

This level focuses on practicing Reiki on others, as well as more advanced energy channeling options. Additionally, students will be taught how to receive Reiki symbols and will also learn the attunement for the second level. The Reiki symbols will let the practitioner connect to the universal energy more deeply and learn all that it can provide to patients. This level also includes the basics of distance Reiki, which means sending healing energy to people no matter where they are.

Due to the intense concentration that these sessions require, level two training can take anywhere from a few weeks to a few months depending on the mental fortitude of the student. Students are typically shown the way to the second level of attunement in a single session focusing on an even wider area of the main channel, with special focus placed on using the heart chakra.

Reiki Level 3

Level 3 is normally thought of as the "teacher's level." The Master blending, along with its symbol is received by many, but they are not comfortable in the proper attunement of others. This is why there is a difference between Master and Third Degree.

The Calm Morning Mind (5 minutes).

This meditation is best in the morning. Choose a nice quiet place where you will not be interrupted. Sit with your legs crossed and back straight, while dropping your head and closing your eyes.

Begin by breathing in slowly, taking a full deep breath and then breathing out slowly and completely as well. Use this time to listen to the signals that your body is providing you with, and try to take them all in as fully as possible.

Focus on breathing and where your breath is going.

Relax your shoulders and feel your whole body relaxing as you do.

Your mind is clearing, moving all thoughts of tasks and stress out, thinking only about the breath that is flowing in and out of your body.

Relax your breathing. Keep breathing slowly in and out.

Think of how your breath is beginning to fill all areas of your body. Moving through your veins and muscles and through your mind as well.

Think of your breath as coolness when it enters your body that is warmed by your body as it leaves. Your body is warming this pure, clean breath.

It fills you as you breathe in and leaves a clearer path behind it.

Breathe easier now. Slow, methodical breaths soothe you.

You are calm. Nothing is in your mind but thoughts of fresh, clean, cool air that enters all parts of your body and brings with it inner peace.

Only think about calm, peace and spiritual love.

You are nourishing your body with love.

Only thoughts of happiness and good health are allowed to reside in you.

Your mind is peaceful. This results in a quiet and gentle mind that takes care of you.

Keep the flow of the air moving in and out of your body and mind, filling every empty space.

Completely relax until you have a feeling of weightlessness. A spiritual feeling. A loving feeling.

Nothing is allowed here but peace... calm... love...

Breathe in...

Breathe out...

You feel completely free and now begin to smell that fresh coffee aroma. You are cleansed and ready to take on all of the positive things the day will bring!

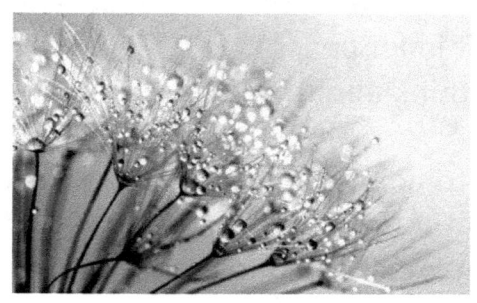

Chapter 5: An Energy By Any Other Name

Is Still The Same

The story of Reiki, as you have read, is ancient and dates back farther than mankind. Our discoveries of it through various cultures and religious concepts and ideas has crossed many lands and periods of our evolution. The basic origins of Reiki are now known to you, and it would still not be fully told if you weren't able to see some of the other possibilities of how Universal life-force finds its way into our cultural identities.

There are many more ways that we have learned about the presence of this light energy and as you go forward through this journey of learning the healing art of Reiki, it is important that you look at some of the other names for it as you grow in your own knowledge and practice.

Ki, Chi, Prana, Light, Kundalini

The term for Reiki comes from the conjunction of the words Rei, meaning

"Universal Life", and Ki, meaning "energy". Reiki is really just a name given by one man who was of Japanese origin and developed his model for channeling this energy to heal others. The combination of these words basically describes the words "Universal life-force" that you have read about already in these pages.

So then, the philosophy of Reiki may be from one cultural background, developed from another cultural background and named in the language of the originator of these techniques and tools, but that name for Universal energy can be found in many other Eastern cultures and practices and it is important to understand that there really is no separation between any of it; just alternative methods for utilizing Universal life-force.

To be clear, Universal life-force (let's call it ULF) is the electrical light vibration and frequency that is humming and pulsing in all matter and all living things. It exists everywhere, in everyone and everything, since the dawn of the cosmic forces we were all born to eons ago. It doesn't matter who is talking about it, or how it works, or what the best way to describe it and utilize it is; it's really all the same essential energy and life-force material that Dr. Usui was able to put into a very easy method of healing approach.

It is important that you understand as many versions of this ULF as possible so that you can understand that the only difference in these names, and the way that they are explained, is cultural belief, philosophy, value and practice.

Ki and Chi (Qi)

As you just learned, Ki in Japan means "life-force", or energy. Ki also has many other translations and contexts, but in the context of healing and the spirit, it means life-force. In China, the word Qi, pronounced Chi, means something along the lines of "vital energy" and is often described in the traditional Chinese medicine doctrines that continue to be powerful for healing methods in the Chinese culture. Chi is described as being a part of everyone, and this living energy requires daily balance and an attitude of moderation and healthy applications in order to stay in alignment with your vitality and strength. The use of healing diets, meditations, certain exercises and herbal remedies are what help this culture maintain their concept and belief of ULF. As with Reiki and the more Buddhist origins of the nature of these concepts, Chi has equally ancient roots and belief systems that support them.

Additionally, the foundation of the physical, meditative arts of Tai Chi and Chi Gong are connected to the ideas and concepts of how to heal, and keep healthy, the Chi, or ULF.

Prana

In the Hindu traditions of India, the ULF is referred to in their religious and spiritual texts as "prana". The literal translation of prana is "life force" and according to their sacred manuscripts, it describes the flow and movement of a person's vital energy through the sections of mind, body and spirit. Various kinds of yoga, the principles of Ayurveda, tantra and other healing techniques, base everything on the balance and wholeness of individual prana, for the ultimate goal of collective wholeness and life force energy flow.

The practices of the Hindu culture and Indian societies may have different applications tending to the ULF, with different names and structures for healing and balance, and they also are greatly linked to the life-force principles of the cultural explanations described as Ki and Qi.

Light

The word "light" has become another popular way to describe ULF. If you look at many of the Christian texts and religions of the world, they often describe the "light of the lord" or the "light of the Holy Spirit," and so on.

Light is not always about Christian faith, either. Many of the doctrines of the yoga practices that have come to our Western culture have used the term to offer a different attitude or description to the work that you do to maintain and balance your inner energy. Light is the highest form of vibration and so, as we seek to attain our greatest frequency, wholeness and health, we seek to become lighter and freer of lower vibrating, or darker flowing energies.

All of these names for ULF are describing the same, essential essence of being. It is present in everyone and all matter, and we have to understand that you can call it whatever you want, but it will always be the same, no matter where you live and what your cultural beliefs are. The name is Universal.

Kundalini

The concept of Kundalini dates back to when the Vedas were being written thousands of years ago. The sacred and ancient Sanskrit documents describe the Kundalini as the life force that lives within you, at the base of your spine, and can only be sparked through ascension and spiritual awakening caused by the opening of the first, or root chakra. The chakras were termed in these texts and are a large part of the way the Hindu cultures discuss healing and prana through the awakening of the true soul power of the individual.

This awakening is often called Kundalini Rising, or Kundalini Awakening and is specific to the culture from whence it came, however the reality is that it can happen to anyone, anywhere, anytime. People all over and across cultures have described spontaneous awakening and didn't have a name to describe it or understand what was happening. There are a lot of online articles currently that talk a lot about the symptoms of this experience and what it feels like when you are going through it.

Essentially, it is the forcing open of the dormant life force that sets in motion an entire cascading opening of every chakra in your body over time, releasing and purging emotional blockages, outworn and outdated life patterns and belief systems, and whatever stands in the way of your pure light and wholeness. This can be a terrifying experience if you don't know what it is, where it came from, or why it is happening in the first place.

Some people purposefully manifest this kind of awakening by utilizing certain kinds of yoga techniques, specifically called Kundalini Yoga, as well as other methods and modalities. Not surprisingly, the healing art of Reiki has been known to spark some awakening, setting the off the energy of the body to shift, purge, cleanse and rebalance over a period of long and challenging personal growth and Reiki therapy work.

Kundalini and Reiki are not the same thing, and yet they inspire similar results. We are all looking for ways to help ourselves feel whole, light, love, joy, balance and mental/emotional/physical health. The quality of these experiences that open you up to energetically purifying yourself on all levels come from the ancient questions and answers that were already being studied well before Dr. Usui developed Reiki.

The chakra system is important to understand as you get more acquainted with Reiki and how it heals the body. Despite the concepts of chakras coming from the Vedas and the Hindu religions, they are a large part of what Dr. Usui programmed into his teachings. He was, after all, a student of Buddha, who referred to such concepts and ideas in his teachings as well.

It makes sense that there would be many cultural bridges to understanding our universal energy and life force. Reiki work can inspire awakening (Kundalini Rising) because of how it shifts and rebalances your energy. This may not always happen for everyone, however, if it is your goal to become more awakened and open through Reiki, you may find that it will look and feel a lot like a total life change and personal growth overture.

Universal Wholeness

What comes from all of these different points of view and concepts of healing and personal power is this one thing: we are all the one whole life force. The power of each of us is great and no matter what we call the ULF in all of us and all life, we have to recognize that underneath all of the borders, backgrounds and beliefs, it is Universal energy and it is all of us.

Within the reality of Reiki, I will be teaching about the concepts of Universal life force and how it can be opened and channeled for healing and more. There isn't any structure to the reality of using this powerful energy; Reiki is a set of principles, pillars, symbols and tools to help you conduct this energy through you and into the body of another to help them transform their energy into its original state of light and vibrational frequency.

When you receive a Reiki treatment, you are not being "healed" by the Master or the practitioner; they are not the ones in control of your light. Reiki is guiding the healing process directly through the practitioner, locating the energetic needs and imbalances in order to figure out the best way to move, transform, release, purge and purify, so that you can live in harmony with yourself and the energy of all things.

The next chapter will spend more time giving information about the chakra system and how it works, why it should be understood for practicing Reiki, and the best ways to connect with your own chakras for healing purposes.

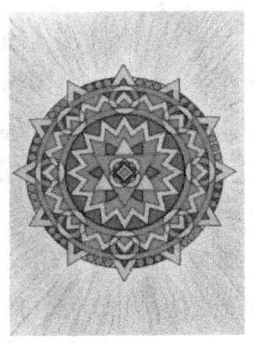

Chapter 6: Establishing Your Intent

Many people who practice Reiki eventually learn to hold it in a high, spiritual regard. This is especially true of those who follow traditional Japanese Reiki, which emphasizes the flow of a spiritual energy and wisdom of a higher power. In order for Reiki to be successful for you, it is crucial that you believe that it will work. Once you have accepted it as a viable means of bringing positivity and healing into your life, you are ready to set your intent for the specific session.

First, however, a little bit of information about why it is so important to clearly set your intent.

Think of the mind as a magnet. When you think passionately about something, the mind attracts what you think of most. If you think negative thoughts and allow the obstacles of life to get you down, you will have a much more negative outlook on life. If you think positively, the things that are positive will come to you. The way to establish what you expect of your Reiki practice is to clearly set your intention beforehand in order to establish the feeling of the life energy that will flow. This chapter will teach you how to do just that.

Technique #1: Namaste

To use this technique, you must get into a bowing position. Place your hands so they are located in the center of your chest, near the heart. Then, close your eyes and slowly bow the head downward. While in this position, ask for Reiki to flow through you, either silently or out loud. After asking for the Reiki to flow, state what you want out of the session. For example, "I set the intent that this session will bring more positivity in my life" or "I set the intent that this session will ease my chronic pain."

Technique #2: Opening Your Palms to the Heavens

If you are asking for guidance from a higher power or want to reach out to the spiritual realms to channel Reiki energy, then you can set the mood for your healing session by opening your palms up to the Heavens. Outstretch your arms in front of your body with the palms up. Raise them until they are above your head and visualize the Reiki flowing from above you into your palms. From there, focus on it coursing from your palms to the rest of your body, filling you with energy. As you feel this energy, take a moment to set your intent for the session.

Technique #3: State Your Intent

Another option for setting your intent is simply stating what you wish to be true. For example, you may say "I set the intent that the anxiety will be removed from my body" or "I set the intent that this session will help clear my mind." State this clearly, firmly, and loudly and pay attention to the way that your intent resonates through your body.

A Few Tips for Setting Your Intention

Tip #1: Be Specific

Imagine that you are using a Reiki session to clear your mind and channel positive energy before you give a presentation at work. Instead of saying "I set the intent that positive energy will flow and mind my mind will be clear," make your session specific to your presentation. Instead, say "I set the intent that my mind will be clear and my body will be full of positive energy instead of anxiety as I give my presentation."

Tip #2: Add "Or Better" to the End of Your Intent

Sometimes, the world has something bigger planned for us then we know. As a result, you may sell yourself short when you set your intentions. To stop yourself from putting limits on the benefits that you will receive, add "or better" at the end of your intention.

Step #3: Avoid Saying What You Don't Want

One common mistake that people make when setting their intent is saying what they don't want. This is incredibly ineffective.

Imagine that you suffer from depression and you are having a particularly bad day. The wrong way to set your intention would be to say, "I don't want to be depressed today." The right way, on the other hand, is to say, "I would like positive vibes to flow through my body and rid it of my depression." Always say what you do want, rather than what you do not want.

Tip #4: Make Sure Your Actions Coincide with Your Intentions

If you do not behave in a way that allows your intentions to manifest, then it is very unlikely you will have success in your ventures.

Imagine that you are trying to rid your mind of anxiety before a big presentation. After performing your Reiki session, you drink 2 large cups of coffee. You are jittery instead of relaxed during your presentation and stumble of your words. In this case, the reason that the healing session did not work is because your actions did not align with the intentions of Reiki.

Surroundings and Timing

Reiki will be most beneficial when performed in a quiet, calm setting. It should also be practiced around the same time each day. For some people, the most beneficial time to do Reiki is first thing in the morning. You do not even have to get out of bed to do it and it helps set the tone for the rest of your day. For others, however, they benefit the most from doing it at night. This is particularly helpful for people with chronic pain or anxiety, who may need a little help sleeping at night.

Think about your specific condition and the time that you think it may be most beneficial. If you choose, you may even practice Reiki more than once a day, as often as you need it. Once you do choose a time for your practice, keep it consistent from day to day. This will give you the best results.

Now that you have set your intention, you are ready to move on to the actual practice of Reiki. Continue to the next chapter to learn more.

Chapter 7: The Human Energy Body

Every cell in the physical human body has a still light energy in it. However, surrounding the physical body is another body of energy known as the Aura or the Human Energy Body. This Aura is made of finer and lighter vibrations. Just as we have different fingerprints, so also each person's auric energy has its own distinctive energy signature.

There are seven energy centers on the human energy body known as chakras and a range of energy channels known as the meridians.

The aura of most people is oval in shape (elliptical) aura, which is fairly larger at the back than at the front, and slightly narrow at the sides, and it also stretches above the head and below the feet. A person's aura is not always the same size. The aura is dependent on a number of factors like how physically and emotionally fit you are and how well suited you are in your environment.

The aura around a person can go up to 2m or even farther away from the physical body. So if you are in the midst of people, this means that your auras are mingling. This also means that your aura precedes you. So you are able to sense things before being physically present.

Also, aura is only present on living things and it's said that its energy is able to pass through dense physical matter. The energies of your aura appear to be either positive or negative depending on its vibrations.

Chakra means a wheel or a vortex. Energy centers around the human body are known as chakras. There are seven chakras located at;

The base of the spine/perineum,
Near the navel,
At the solar plexus,
In the middle of the chest,
In the throat,
In the center of the brow,
At the crown of the head.

I strongly recommend you read my book on Chakra for beginners before you take on this course.

Each of these chakras is connected to specific parts of the body. So when a particular chakra is healthy and without damage, the related parts of the body are seen to be healthy as well. But when a chakra is damaged, blocked or torn, the corresponding parts of the body are generally unwell. Like our aura, the chakras are also subject to being affected by a divergent number of factors like physical and emotional wellness as well as environmental factors.

The meridians are the channels through which auric energy flows. They carry our 'ki' around to all parts of the body. The major meridians are line longitudinally along the body.

The Human Energy Body and Health

Like we have clearly established above, there is a marked relationship between the state of our energy body and our overall state of physical wellness.

Everything we come in contact with is capable of positively or negatively affecting our auras. The people we talk to, the things we laugh at, the things we read, the things we smell, the way we laugh, the things we eat, the things we think and say – everything we do.

Everything that we interact with can change our aura. The more negative these things are, the more they lower our energy body vibrations. However, as we experience positive things or things that make us happy, our positive energy vibrations increases thereby forming a balance.

The amount of ki found within us is not constant. It varies from day to day. Our body soaks up ki from all around us to serve the same deficit. From the food we eat for example, the more ki we have within us, the more natural healing power we possess.

Ki is the natural energy in and around all things. Reiki is the specific energy on a particular frequency that is released from the Source for healing. What this means is that Reiki, unlike ki, does not naturally flow through everyone and everything. It only flows through people who have been spiritually empowered or attuned to its spiritual frequency.

Since Reiki is an irreligious technique, it is made available to all and sundry irrespective of tribe, race, creed, intellectual capacity and personal belief system. No special skill is required. One only needs to attend Reiki First Class degree and receive the attunement.

Reiki Energy as a Healing Treatment

The process of Reiki healing technique is quite simplistic. The recipient either lies on a massage table or sits. Whichever way, they are often advised to take their shoes off. There is no elaborate ritual to the process.

A simple intention to use Reiki is enough to get flowing. The spiritually attuned person then places his or her hands gently on the head or any other part of the body that needs healing and holds still or taps very gently.

Reiki healing works from the inward and then projects to the outward. As energy flows into the aura and the body, chakras are being cleared and properly balanced and meridians are being strengthened and straightened to their optimum. The inflow of energy revitalizes the body's natural healing ability. As Reiki is guided by a higher influence, the healing energy is able to go into the body and precisely flow to the places that need healing the most without any guidance from the recipient or the Reiki Master. This energy is also self-regulatory so the patient never takes in more or less than they actually need — they get just enough.

This healing is almost instantaneous in some cases as it harmonizes and balances the physical body. It is important to note that Reiki on its own does not heal. What it does is to condition and activate your body's natural healing ability to heal itself. This means that response to Reiki often differs. One condition may take longer to heal than another. It also implies that it works differently from person to person.

So, 5 people, for example, with similar symptoms who subject themselves to Reiki will experience 5 different outcomes depending on the recipient's mental, physical and emotional state.

Reiki healing starts within as earlier mentioned, so even though you may be manifesting physical symptoms, it may have to heal you emotionally first. However, if Reiki healing must remain permanent for you, you may have to focus on healing the root cause.

The Physical Healing Process

Healing is the restorative process of good health from a damaged, unbalanced or diseased state. Our bodies have an innate healing ability that is able to repair and maintain itself by cell growth and division. The replacement can happen in two ways; either regeneration or by repair. Regeneration is when the necrotic cells are replaced by new cells that form "like" tissue – as was originally there, while repair is one in which injured tissues are replaced with scar tissue. Many organs in the body heal by the combination of these two processes.

The steady replication and repair of cells is what makes physical healing possible. Again, this healing ability is dependent on a number of factors like what you eat, what you drink, how emotionally stable you are and so forth.

Healing does not happen in abstract. It doesn't happen out there or out-of-body, it comes from within. It is only you who is capable of healing yourself. Your body has been built in a way that makes it possible for it to heal itself. The most that anyone can do for you is to kick-start that natural process.

The pertinent question to ask here is that if the body is self-healing, why then do people suffer from incurable diseases? It is because healing is a holistic process and not a merely physical one. A number of factors could be responsible for incurable or cancerous illnesses. It could be that the emotional state of the patient is not very healthy or that the immune system has been severely damaged as a result of some earlier stressful event. If the body is able to return back to its normal balanced state, it will be able to fight off those diseases even without medical intervention.

Healing can occur on different levels:

On a physical level, where the physical symptoms can be stopped or at least limited

On an emotional level, where fears are confronted

On a mental level, and

On a spiritual level.

Healing as a whole are categorized into three distinct models:

The Biomedical model

This is a purely physical perspective to healing. It views the body as a separate entity, unable to be influenced by the mind or emotions. This is conventional medicine, where the body is seen as a system and any illness is seen a mere malfunction of one of its components. It involves treatments via chemicals, radiations, surgery, etc.

The Holistic model

This healing model treats not just the symptoms but also the causes of an ailment. Not only will the physical body get treated, the mind and other related aspects of the body are also being treated as well. It assumes that any physical ailment is a direct consequence of a state of mental or emotional unwellness. So if the underlying cause is not treated, the disease cannot be healed or the symptoms may be treated and may go away temporarily but ultimately, the person will fall ill again.

Treatments such as osteopathy, chiropractic, acupuncture, homeopathy, aromatherapy, reflexology and healing techniques such as Reiki all fall into this category.

The metaphysical model

Here, everything is seen as energy. Metaphysical healers aim to correct the disassociation between body and mind. Treatments such as chakra balancing, unblocking and healing deal in revitalizing the body by redirecting the body's energy.

Chapter 8: Getting Started

The first thing that you need to familiarize yourself with would be the different hand positions as this is what you'll need in order to get the healing process started. There are two kinds. One is for self-healing, and the other for healing others. They are both quite easy to learn so you'll be able to focus more on directing your energy when performing any of the two healing methods.

During a typical session, you will need to place your hands on the different locations for at least 3 to 5 minutes at a time. You can also extend the time and simply depend upon your intuition. Make sure that your hands are slightly cupped and that your fingers are close together. Remember that the lighter your touch is, the better it will be.

Remember that intention is the most important factor that determines the success of a treatment. Pray or focus your intentions towards the patient and ask for the highest level of healing, making you a channel for Reiki energy. The healing isn't from you but works through you.

Reiki Hand Positions for Self-Treatment:

First Position (Face) – Place the palms of your hands against your face with your hands slightly cupped over your eyes. Lightly touch your fingers upon your forehead while you do this as well.

Second Position (Crown and top of the head) - Place both of your hands on each side of your head, making sure that the heels of your hands are resting right near your ears with your fingertips touching the crown of your head.

Third Position (Side of the head) - Place each of your hands on each side of your head just directly on each ear and temple.

Fourth Position (Back of the head) – Cross your arms behind your head while placing one hand on the back of it and resting the other directly above your nape. An alternative is placing both hands at the back of the head then do the nape after.

Fifth Position (Chin and jaw line) – Cup your hands and rest it under your chin, allowing your fingers to wrap along your jaw line.

Sixth Position (Neck, collarbone, and heart) – Lightly grasp your neck in the throat area using the V shape formed by your thumb and fingers. Lower your other hand slowly, resting it between your collarbone and heart center.

Seventh Position (Shoulder blades) – Slowly reach over your head, bending your elbows comfortably while you place both hands on your shoulder blades. However, if you can't do this with ease, just place your hands over your shoulders and that should serve the same purpose.

Eighth Position (Ribs and ribcage or upper stomach) – Gently place both hands on top of your upper ribcage, which is right below your breasts. Make sure that your bent elbows are relaxed.

Ninth Position (Abdomen or middle stomach) – Place your hands on your tummy between the solar plexus and the area above the navel. Make sure your fingertips are touching when you do so.

Tenth Position (Pelvic bones or lower stomach) – Over each pelvic bone, place one of your hands. Again, make sure that your fingertips are touching each other and that you use minimal pressure on the area.

Eleventh Position (Middle back) – Reach behind your back once more with both elbows bent while you put both hands on the center of your back.

Twelfth Position (Lower back) – For this, you have to reach behind again with elbows bent then slowly put both hands on your lower back area. Do this carefully so you don't end up pulling a muscle.

Thirteenth Position (Knees) – Sit down on a chair or an exercise floor mat or a firm mattress where you can reach each bended knee with a hand. As an alternative you can do it one knee at a time placing one hand on the knee cap (top) and the other on the knee joint (below).

Fourteenth Position (Left foot) – Sit down on an exercise floor mat or firm mattress where you can stretch the right leg and bend the left leg flat on the surface. Place each hand on the top and bottom part of the left foot.

Fifteenth Position (Right foot) — Now do things inversely on the right foot. Maintain the sitting position, but this time stretch the left leg, and bend the right leg. Then place each hand on the top and bottom part of the right foot.

Sixteenth Position (Right and left heel of both feet) — Maintaining the seated position, bend both legs flat on the surface then hold the heel of each foot with a hand. Left hand to the left heel, and right hand to the right heel.

Aside from all these positions (see corresponding 16 illustrations on the succeeding page), you may add or include those portions of your body where you're experiencing a discomfort, fatigue, stiffness, pain or even a diagnosed ailment. For example, if you have breathing problems then place your hands on your chest or lung area. Do the corresponding hand position when you have problems on your upper arm (biceps or triceps), elbow, forearm, wrist, crotch, thigh, lower leg, etc. You can have one hand placed on a body part or both hands. If your hand has a problem, place the good hand on it. Even if both hands are not well, you can still use one hand on the other alternately. Or you can also ask someone else to heal your hands. To have an idea on how this works, refer to the hand positions for healing others.

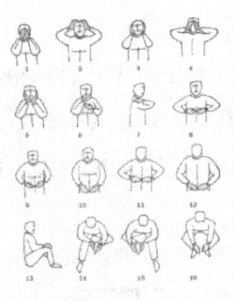

Reiki Hand Positions for Healing Others:
Essentially the things you learned about treating yourself using the various hand positions from head to foot will be used to your patient. You can add more positions especially those body parts where your

patient is feeling some pain or ailment. Make your patient relax in a seated or lying position. Just let your patient adjust sides or turn over when doing some positions like the back. As a guide, you may follow these for the sequence:

Head (Stand by the top of the patient's head) - crown, under the head, eyes, jaw, ears, neck, and the collar bone.

Arms (Start with the right before moving to the left part) - shoulder, upper arm, elbow, wrist, hand, and fingers.

Trunk - upper chest, breast area, ribs, lower abdomen, first "V-shaped" hand position instead of "T" to the groin area, waist, then "T-shaped" hand position back to the upper chest.

Legs (begin from the right then move to the left) – thigh, knee, lower leg, ankles, the arch of the foot, and the toes.

Back (best done if you have your patient lie on their stomach) – do the "V" position at base of the spine and the "T" to the shoulders. Remember to start at the shoulders while criss-crossing your hands as you move down the spine and the buttocks.

As an added tip and aid when performing these hand positions especially to others is the use of beautiful Reiki music. This is to better relax the mind and minimize distractions. You can find FREE Reiki music for healing, meditation, well-being, and relaxation in the internet sites like YouTube. Here you can find not just music specifically for Reiki but also powerful symbols and tutorial guides to performing the hand positions.

Be warned though that there will always be rude critics in the comments section even on those well-produced videos. Naturally, it's understandable to have these negative comments if the video is not professionally done. It's so easy to judge it as quack if the video is executed poorly. So choose what you listen to and/or watch. And since Reiki is also an alternative method of healing, not all people would easily believe, understand, try, or appreciate it. The key is having an open mind, if not a positive belief, when trying Reiki. For only then will the positive healing energy flow and do its work. A carefully chosen music and/or video will help relax the mind and the rest of the body. Same goes to having a comfortable bed, chair, or mat in a room with just the right relaxing lighting, scent, and temperature.

Chapter 9: The History Of Reiki

In the Footsteps of DR MIKAO USUI (1865-1926)

The founder of the Usui Shiki Ryoho, the Reiki Healing System, was Dr. Mikao Dr Usui, a Japanese Buddhist lecturer who later taught at the Tokyo University in the theological seminary. Dr Usui was born on the 15**th** of August 1865 in the village of Taniai (now called Miyama cho) in the Yamagata country of the Gifu Prefecture in Japan. He died less than a hundred years ago on 9 March 1926. Today Dr Usui's name can be found carved on a huge torii (literally 'bird abode') gate at the entrance of the Shinto Amataka Shrine close to where his home once stood. A traditional Japanese torii symbolically marks the changeover from the profane to the sacred.

It is surprising how few written and recorded facts exist about Dr Usui as a person. This may partially be to the fact that many documents were lost during

World War II. Besides, most of the people whom he knew and whom he taught are either unknown or no more alive. This great lack of documentation and recorded material about him, has unfortunately led to many myths and speculations growing around his life, thus converting sometimes Reiki history into Reiki fiction.

However, based on whatever little records remain about Dr Usui's life, it is believed that Dr Usui sensei came from a wealthy family. The reason for this belief is that during those years, only children from wealthy families could get good schooling, tutoring and education.

Even if the exact dates of Dr Usui's schooling and higher education years remain uncertain, it is believed that Dr Usui received his Reiki ingenuity and ability around the 1914s. This belief has been supported by works from former great Reiki Masters, among whom Hyakuten Inamoto, Japanese Buddhist monk and Founder of the Komyo Reiki Kai style of Reiki. Inamoto was a former student of Mrs.. Chiyoko Yamaguchi who was herself a direct student of Dr Usui's student, Dr Chujiro Hayashi. According to written records, Dr Usui carried out for 21 days a rigid fasting and meditation on Mt. Kurama (Kurama-yama). This exercise was a strict practice called 'Discipline of Prayer and Fasting' prevalent among great monks and sages of those days. It is believed that on the 21st day, the last day of his meditation and fasting, Dr Usui Mikao attained enlightenment and experienced the Reiki phenomenon.

The Usui Reiki Years

According to available records, it is believed that Dr Usui began his 3-year Zen training in the 1918-1919 years. An article written in 1928 by Shou Matsui, a student of Dr Chujiro Hayashi (student of Dr Usui) reveals: "It has been more than ten years since Reiki Ryoho was founded." This revelation leads us to believe that Dr Usui might have started teaching Reiki to his students and patients earlier than 1922 which is the commonly accepted period.

It is also supposed that by 1921 Dr Usui began working as a secretary of Gotō

Shinpei, a statesman and cabinet minister in the Taishō and early Shōwa period Empire of Japan. According to same sources, it was in these years that Dr Usui apparently incorporated the 'Five Ideals' or 'Five Principles of Reiki' into his teachings.

After attaining the Reiki Experience on Mt. Kurama, Dr Usui is said to have practised Reiki on himself and on members of his family first before starting to teach Reiki to people and offer healing sessions to them. Many claim that the teachings of Dr Usui are of Buddhist origin. His teachings are also said to have included Shinto energy practices. In fact, it is also claimed that Dr Usui's Reiki originates from Gautam Buddha. Usui did not even name his Healing System. It was then referred to as the Usui-Do or the Usui Way.

It is believed that Dr Usui opened his very first dojo (training hall) in Harajuku, Tokyo. The dojo is what we would call a 'clinic' in the modern day. According to beliefs it was during these times that Dr Usui also founded the Usui Reiki Healing Method

Learning Society. Dr Usui's motto was: 'Unity of Self through Harmony and Balance.'

On September 1, 1923, a 7.9 earthquake struck Yokohama and Tokyo. The death reported was over 140,000. Dr Usui and his students helped in the healing of rescued victims in the area. His Healing practice grew into great prominence during this tragedy.

On March 9, 1926, Dr Usui died at the age of 62 in Fukuyama town. He had suffered a massive stroke. He was buried in Saihoji Temple, in Tokyo.

Dr Chujiro Hayashi (1880 – 1940)

Dr Usui's met with Dr Chujiro Hayashi in the mid 20s and became his student. Hayashi, who was born in Tokyo on Sept 15, 1880, was a physician in the Japanese naval army.

As there was no war during those times, Dr Hayashi was on leave and had specially come to Tokyo with the purpose of learning Reiki from Dr Usui. He was interested in the Usui technique of healing without medical drugs.

Dr Hayashi thought this technique would be of great help to soldiers in times of war. Dr Usui welcomed Dr Hayashi in his Training Center and taught him Reiki. After acquiring his Reiki Mastership, Dr Hayashi, however, did not return to the Navy. Instead, he continued working with Dr Usui. In fact, he not only joined Dr Usui's Centre but remained with Dr Usui until the death of the Master. Later, as per Dr Usui's wish, Dr Chujiro Hayashi took complete charge of Dr Usui's clinic after the latter's death, for he had promised not to let the miraculous healing technique be lost forever to the world.

A few months after Dr Usui's death, Dr Hayashi moved the Usui Reiki Training Center to Shina-no-Machi in Tokyo.

By 1930, Dr Hayashi started reforming his system which was still almost entirely based on Dr Usui's teachings and principles. It was named the Hayashi Reiki Ryoho Kenkyukai. In 1931, Chujiro Hayashi left the Gakkai because he was unhappy with the then Naval Officers' nationalistic attitudes. Nonetheless, he continued to teach the Usui-Do together with his own System.

Mrs Hawayo Takata (1900-1980)

In 1935, another person entered the Usui Reiki Ryoho scene in Japan in the person of Hawayo Kawamuru Takata, born in Kauai, Hawaii, on December 24, 1900. Takata's parents were Japanese who, like hundreds of others in those days, had migrated to Hawaii as indentured laborers to work in the sugarcane fields. Hawayo grew up and married Saichi Takata, also a laborer, and were blessed with two children, both girls.

However, life became arduous for Hawayo after she lost her 34 year old husband in October 1930. Work was daunting in the fields but she had no other choice but to toil hard in order to feed her children. A year later Hawayo found her health declining rapidly. She had excruciating pain in the abdomen which, she was told by her doctor, needed immediate surgery. To top it all she also suffered from asthma which made it difficult for her to breathe. Hawayo was only 35 at that time, but, as she later said it herself, she looked 60. She hardly had any money to afford surgery in the US. Hawayo was finally compelled to ask for help from her paternal family in Japan who replied that they could not afford to send her so much money abroad for the simple reason that they did not have it. Instead they sent her a ticket saying she could come to Japan and undergo surgery in one of the hospitals in Tokyo and that they would take care of her.

Hawayo left for Japan alone leaving her two daughters with her sister Kauwayo. Upon her arrival in Tokyo, she was immediately admitted in a hospital where medical tests diagnosed a cancerous tumor in her abdomen. However, according the doctors, Hawayo's asthmatic condition could pose a severe problem during surgery as chloroform was the only anesthetic in those years. The doctor knew there was little hope for Hawayo if any. Nevertheless, at the time she was getting ready to be taken to the operation theater, Hawayo heard an inner voice telling her: 'You are not in need of surgery, Hawayo; you'll get healed naturally...'

Hawayo Takata said later that she heard this voice again and again and so clearly that she could no longer ignore it. She spoke to the surgeon who was getting ready to put her to sleep. But strangely enough it was this surgeon who advised Hawayo to go try her luck at the next-door Reiki clinic which was run at that time by Dr Chujiro Hayashi.

Dr Hayashi and Takata Team for the Cause of Reiki

Hawayo Takata was not only admitted but was welcome at the clinic of Dr Hayashi who immediately started healing sessions on her. Hawayo, not having enough money to meet the cost of her treatment, offered to work free of charge at the clinic for Dr Hayashi if ever her health was restored.

Few months of intensive Reiki treatment at Dr Hayashi's Clinic breathed new life into Hawayo and she was literally brought back to life. She soon got herself back on the road to health. Her tumor had disappeared and she had no more breathing problems. When she was completely healed and rehabilitated, she started working for Dr Hayashi at the Clinic as a helper.

A few months later, Takata moved into Dr Hayashi's house where she stayed for a long time as an uchideshi or a live-in student and received special training from him. Hawayo took concentrated Reiki classes from Dr Hayashi and was soon healing patients at the Clinic. Dr Hayashi bestowed upon Hawayo the innermost secret of Energy Science, known as the Shinpe Den (the **Master Level of Reiki)**, the Kokiyu-ho (the dry bathing technique) and the Leiji-ho (the intuitive method of finding where to lay the hands on the patient). These were considered as the utmost secrets in the EnergySphere.

In the summer of 1937, Dr Hayashi went with his daughter to Hawaii, where he and Mrs. Takata promoted Reiki Healing through a wide lecture tour.

In February, 1938, Dr Hayashi certified Takata as a Master and a Practitioner of the Dr Usui's Reiki Healing System.

Meanwhile, the Second World War showed no sign of coming to an end. In 1940, Dr Hayashi was summoned by the Naval Army to return to his duty as a soldier. All retired army officers and soldiers were being called back to duty as there was a shortage of young and able soldiers. Dr Hayashi could not refuse. If he did so he would be considered not only an enemy and a coward, but also arrested with court martial and imprisoned. Hayashi was standing at the crossroads, thinking about the long years he had spent healing and helping people of his country. He could not bear the thought of going back to the Army, taking up arms and killing fellow beings.

Hayashi finally made up his mind. He decided to 'make the transition', as he described it to Mrs. Takata who was unable to understand the meaning of his words until the 9**th** of May of 1940. Dr Hayashi had summoned all the Reiki

Masters he had trained and all his students. He explained to them that war between the US and Japan was now inevitable and he knew that many people, including his Reiki Masters and students, would perish sooner or later. He also expressed his apprehension about Reiki being lost forever.

Dr Hayashi also remembered that Dr Usui, in his final days, had taken a pledge from him that whatever happened, he should never let his Healing Technique die off like so many others had done before.

How was Dr Hayashi to keep a promise he had made to Dr Usui when his own end was so near?

It was at that critical juncture—during those obscure days—that Hayashi suddenly came to understand the purpose of Mrs. Takata's presence at the Clinic. He caught the drift of her existence in his surroundings. First, Hawayo was a foreigner; second she had been given a new lease of life through Reiki. Truth finally dawned on Dr Hayashi. This was no coincidence. It was a sign that Reiki was destined to stay, to continue and to spread out as Dr Usui's had wished it. Dr Hayashi was relieved at the thought that he had already given the Mastership Course to Mrs. Takata.

On the fateful day, Dr Hayashi invited all his Masters, students and friends and explained to them the meaning of the word 'transition' which meant that he would soon be leaving his body. But prior to that, he took a promise from Mrs. Takata that she would spend the rest of her life—the new life granted to her by the Divine Energy—promoting the cause of Reiki. He made her promise that she would keep the flame of Reiki burning by continuing on the path of Dr Usui and by carrying on with the Usui Reiki Technique. He told Mrs. Takata that her country—Hawaii—would not be affected by War and Reiki would be safe there and in her hands. Hayashi finally gave Mrs. Takata her all the money and the legal papers of the Clinic and requested her to go back to her country after his death.

At precisely 1 p.m. he called upon his wife, asking her to stay near him and he left this world without pain and in great dignity. Dr Hayashi was 62 and in perfect health when he died. He was incinerated as per the Zen tradition.

Mrs. Takata, abiding by the commands of her late Mentor, accepted the money. But before leaving Japan, she transferred all the assets related to the Clinic and the house to Mrs. Hayashi.

During the war, Dr Hayashi's clinic was turned over to military use, especially as a hospital for war casualties. Many took refuge there during the bombing periods which were regular and almost never-ending. While the whole country was being ruthlessly attacked and death was rained down on the town, one place stood out though, as clear as day and for all to see. Dr Hayashi's clinic miraculously escaped the terror attack and the powerful bombings of World War II. In fact, according to hearsay, the Clinic was the only building which got away clean from being razed to the ground by bombings. Was it because Hayashi's Reiki Clinic was Energy gridded and nothing could affect it? The answer can only be guessed. The Clinic, still stands in perfect condition where it originally stood and is presently the first Reiki Museum in Tokyo to exhibit Dr Usui's personal belongings, his books and his notes.

Hawayo Takata returned to Hawaii, her native land where she played a major role in the preservation, promotion and dissemination of Reiki out of Japan as per the guidance of her great Mentor, Dr Hayashi. Takata succeeded in presenting Reiki to the Western World as Usui Shiki Ryoho and also in turning Reiki into a less mystical practice.

During her lifetime Mrs. Takata trained 22 Reiki Masters who in turn formed others, thus spreading the Usui Reiki Healing System to other countries throughout the world. The result was that by 1970 Reiki had reached the shores of America, Canada and Europe.

Mrs. Takata died in December 1980 at the age of 80.

The Reiki World is today grateful to Mrs. Hawayo Takata for taking Reiki from Japan to the West and for passing it on to millions of people throughout the world where the numbers continue to grow. Had it not been for Takata sensei, the Usui Reiki System would have most likely never seen the day as a wonderful healing system in the West. Without her Reiki would have in all likelihood been confined to a small number of practitioners even in its own country of origin.

As Reiki channels, we have all benefitted from the traditional sequence of events related to the History of Reiki; and this has been reproduced in this book. However, information coming from the West regarding Dr Usui remains very limited. There have been so many versions related to the History of Reiki and to that of Dr Usui's own life, that one wonders which is the most authentic and honest to goodness. However, much still remains to be verified.

It is also widely believed that after the Second World War, Reiki disappeared from Japan, thus leaving Mrs Takata as the only Reiki Teacher and propagator in the whole world. This belief has never been validated or authenticated. In fact, we know today that the 'Usui Shiki Ryoho' has always existed and still exists in Japan. The Usui Technique of Healing may not have been known as Reiki in the earlier days in Japan, but it never disappeared from there.

However, whatever the veracity and the facts, Reiki Channels will always feel and remain deeply connected to Dr Usui and to the roots of the wonderful healing technique he created and handed over to them. Reiki Channels cannot but help being grateful to Dr Hayashi and to Mrs Takata, who made its continued existence possible outside Japan and ultimately in the whole world.

Chapter 10: The Reiki Levels And Attunements

The levels of Reiki are part of the doctrine of the practice originally outlined by Dr. Usui. Each level is a part of the performance of Reiki and what you will be doing with your energy at that degree. The levels are often referred to as degrees and not levels, but you may find it documented both ways if you continue to study Reiki further. When you are "attuned" to Reiki energy by a Master, you are receiving the opening to channel Reiki energy through your hands. This is how you begin to practice Reiki.

There are many people who have explored channeling energy through their hands without first being attuned by a Reiki Master. This is not unheard of and can occur for people who are already experiencing spiritual awakening and living their life in a way that allows them to have a more opened crown chakra. The chakras are one of the main things you will learn about when you are working with Reiki because the chakras are the channel that Reiki will flow through.

In **Chapter 5: The Science of Reiki**, you will learn more about the chakras and why they are so important, as well as the auric field and how using Reiki flow will also impact the health of the auras and their ongoing wellness in your life.

The Reiki levels are as follows:

First Degree

In the first degree of Reiki, the student is opened to the Universal life force energy by the Reiki Master through the first degree Reiju, or attunement. This attunement is what opens your life-force channel so that you can begin to feel the energy of Reiki in the palms of your hands. This energy may be the most subtle to start with, and with practice will strengthen and become more consistent.

Some students have described the initial sensation in the palms of the hands as being tingling, warm, humming, magnetic, or buzzing. It varies for every person and can depend a lot on how open that person is already as a channel. There are a lot of ways that the first degree can spark a practice of spiritual awakening because it teaches you to work on yourself frequently and help your own energy healing. You are also able to work on other people with the first level attunement and you will connect to yourself more strongly at this time, with this degree of Reiki.

Many people will begin to feel a lot of personal healing and shift as they begin to channel the energy through their hands and into specific parts of the body. As you learn more about the chakras you will understand more about why they are used to help guide and direct the hand placements around your body as a way to help specific ailments or needs.

Also, in the first level of Reiki, you are taught the foundation of Dr. Usui's principles. You will learn the origins and history, as well as the pillars and principles so that you are familiar with the Reiki practice in general. As you read through this book, you will have a better knowledge of Reiki the way you would in instruction for the first degree of Reiki from a Master teacher.

Second Degree

In the second degree of Reiki, you learn a great deal more and are introduced to what is known as the Reiki symbols. The Reiki symbols were a part of the recorded story of Usui's original epiphany of what Reiki is and how to use it. The symbols introduced themselves to him through a vision and he was able to understand what they meant and how to bring them into usual practice.

In the second attunement from the master teacher you are learning from, your channels are further opened and you will feel and even stronger vibration of energy in the palms of your hands. This energy is how Reiki acts through you. You are the conduit of energy to pass through the palms and connect to another energy, either that of your own chakras and auras, or someone else whom you are working on.

In the first degree, you are shown simple methods to use on yourself and other people. A series of hand positions are often taught by the master and these hand positions are usually directly linked to the position of the chakras. Once you are more familiar with where each chakra is located, all you have to do is gently cup the hands, either touching the body above the chakra or hovering an inch or two above the chakra. You don't actually have to touch someone for Reiki to work. Level Two Reiki is often what is used for those who are choosing to become practitioners either more professionally, or to heal more people in their close circle of family and friends.

The symbols are a major part of healing with others, although they are as useful in any treatments you will perform on yourself. The symbols are as follows:

The Power Symbol:

The power symbol, known as Cho Ku Rei, is used the most often for a specific reason: any time you draw the other two symbols, you will draw the power symbol before and after. It is basically the light switch for healing, opening the pathways with the self or anyone else you may be treating. This symbol can be used for purifying and cleansing energy as well as in the protection of spaces, like your home, car, and other areas.

The Mental Symbol:

This symbol, Sei Heiki, is what is used mainly for mental and emotional issues and blockages in the auras and chakras. It will often be used in treatments where someone has a lot of emotional upheaval or chronic problems with depression, sadness, anxiety, worry, and so forth. It can be very helpful for relationship issues, as well, and is powerful for helping people with stopping and ending bad habits, like smoking or alcohol addiction.

The Distance Symbol:

The symbol for distance healing is called Hons Sha Ze Sho Nen and is specifically used for healing other people at a distance. This means that you can send Reiki energy to anyone, anywhere on Earth, at any time with their permission.

This symbol is also effective for healing large groups, the environment, disasters like floods and hurricanes, and so forth. It is also used for healing and treating issues from the distant past, including karma from past lives, and will also help create positive life force energy for future events that are yet to occur.

The Sei Heiki and Hon Sha Ze Sho Nen symbols are always drawn with the power symbol, Cho Ku Rei, before and after the symbols are drawn to empower them and bring them to life.

Each of these symbols can be used on the self and others and are the major aspect of the second degree of Reiki. The Reiju (attunement) for the second degree enhances the energy of the Reiki passing through your palms in a big way. The time between first and second-degree attunement is usually at least 21 days. Many Masters will prefer not to attune someone to the second degree until they have had a few weeks to practice Reiki at the first level and allow for some healing change, to experiment with their own healing process.

Third Degree

The third degree of Reiki is when the student becomes the Master and is able to receive the 4th symbol, known as the Master symbol. The Master symbol is what will allow a Master to attune another person to Reiki and so much of what is taught at this level is how to teach and attune new students to the Reiki philosophy and practice. Many people who choose to go to a Master level have been practicing Level Two Reiki for months or sometimes years before they are ready to become a Master. Sufficient practice is required in order to truly understand the power of being a healing channel of light for other people in the world, as well as to teach it.

Usui Tibetan Master Level

The 4th level is a not as commonly taught, but is still considered a level and here is why: there are 4 more Master symbols that are given at this level and when you are becoming attuned by a Master to become a Master it is not unheard of that you would receive these additional symbols at the third degree of attunement. It depends on your Master and what their teaching philosophy is.

The channels are considered to be even further opened at this level, and what is important to note is that the third and fourth levels of Reiki are typically blended into one "Master Level" and taught all at once. There are still those who will separate them and are usually traditionalists to the prescribed "Usui" way of doing things. As Reiki has spread, its teachings have evolved and differed from Master to Master.

Attunements (Reijus)

The Reiki attunements occur at every level and are performed by the Master. He or she will perform a series of motions and breaths to help open your channels to Reiki. The student will usually be seated in a chair while the Master walks around them and draws the Reiki symbols into their palms and the chakras of the body, like the crown, heart, and feet, to 'tune' the energy to be opened to receiving Reiki. The process only takes about 15-20 minutes or less depending on the Master's preferences. A lot of people are taught Reiki in large groups and workshops and are attuned together in a group. If you are learning in a larger class, you will have to wait for your turn to be attuned, so it might take longer because of that.

Once the attunement is completed, you will be able to feel the Reiki energy in the palms of your hands immediately and will have a great shift in your overall energy. You can then start to practice beaming healing light through the crown of your head and through your palms into the places that need healing.

At the first level attunement, you will be mostly just beaming energy from the palms to cleanse the auras and chakras through either holding the hands directly above these areas, until it feels time to move them, or you may be "pulling energy" out of the self or others, that needs to be removed.

Once you are attuned to the second degree and have the symbols to use as healing tools, you will draw symbols in the air over the chakras and auras, as much as you use your hand positions learned in the first degree. With each attunement, the Reiki energy feels stronger and the more you practice with it, the easier and more stable the energy comes forward to perform healing work.

In a nutshell, there are three levels of Reiki and attunement for each one. You can argue that there is a fourth Master level of Reiki, but the third degree is also a Master level and so they are often pushed together into one workshop. Either way, the Master level is where you learn the symbols for attuning and teaching others, and when Reiki becomes more of a way of life than a practice.

In the next chapter, you will move on through the pillars and principles of Reiki as they were taught by Dr. Usui to give you a background and foundation in the philosophy of how to support Reiki healing in your own life journey.

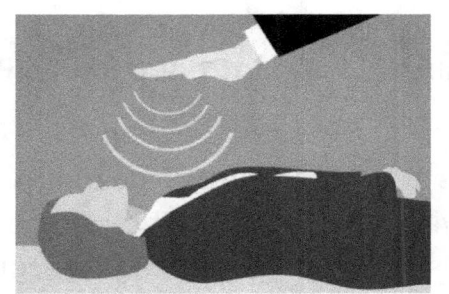

Chapter 11: An Introduction To Reiki

Reiki is the accent art of healing by using the laying on of hands. The person who is administering the healing becomes a vessel for the healing energy addressing physical, mental, emotional and spiritual issues that the recipient is dealing with.

Before we go any further, I want to explain that this can be very dangerous for the person practicing Reiki. When you practice Reiki you have to open yourself up to the healing energies. This can also open you up to many other energies as well. Those who are not experienced can allow negative energies to come into them and although this will not harm the recipient it has been known to cause many issues in the person who is practicing's life.

Many people will tell you that you do not have to worry about protecting yourself when you are practicing but that you need to make sure you are balance. While I do believe that it is very important to be balanced within oneself when practicing

Reiki, I also believe it is important to set up a barrier so that if any negative energy were trying to come your way you would be safe from any harm.

It is just like when a psychic prepares for a session, they know they are going to encounter good but on the off chance any negative comes their way the prepare for it beforehand. You can choose not to protect yourself and that is completely up to you but this next little bit is for those who would like some protection.

The first thing you need to do is choose a spiritual path and follow it. I am not going to get into a discussion on the different paths and opinions on each but you have to understand that Reiki is a very spiritual process therefore you need to ground yourself in a spiritual belief. This does not mean that you have to become a saint over night, what it means is that you try.

Once you have chosen a spiritual path you are going to pray for protection from every negative energy that would try to come against you. While you are healing, if you feel anything negative coming toward you,

you should focus on a sacred object from whatever spiritual path you have chosen.

Finally after the session is over you need to break all ties with any negative energy that may have come upon you.

Many people who practice Reiki inadvertently take on the issues of the person they are healing so if you are healing someone with a mental disorder you need to physically speak out that you break any ties with mental disorders and you do not allow them in your life.

It may seem a little strange at first but you will get used to speaking these things out. And since you are practicing Reiki to begin with you probably already understand they type of havoc negative energy can wreak on a persons life.

You also need to understand that you do not control the healing Reiki energy. Therefore you are going to be unable to tell someone you are going to help them with a specific issue. You see, a person may come to you with a physical issue or you may try to heal yourself of a specific physical issue only to find that it has not been affected. The Reiki energy goes to where it is need most in the body, bringing complete balance.

So if you are going to practice Reiki you need to explain to people that you cannot heal a specific problem but the Reiki energy will heal what is needed the most. It works like this, if someone came into my home and stated that they needed physical healing because they were always tired, the Reiki energy then finds that they are depressed therefore needing mental or emotional healing in order to bring balance to their lives. The Reiki energy would work on the depression and not the symptom of feeling tired.

Often times this discourages people but if it is explained beforehand they tend to be more accepting of the healing no matter what it is.

Chapter 12: The Planes Of Existence

As already mentioned, the names given to these energy-body impressions and planes of existence can vary in number, type and name according to which source the information comes from.

But in general terms, consist of the following:

Physical
Astral
Mental
Intuitional
Spiritual
Monadic
Divine

These seven planes of existence, each have seven sub-divisions which each have seven sub-divisions, which each have seven sub-divisions, which each have...

...and so on, and so on until you reach the seventh sub division of the seventh sub-division.

Quite a lot then, isn't there?

And did you notice something about the number seven? It appeared quite a few times - huh? It's very popular with occultists and the like.

Seven is known as the number of spirituality, sensitivity and mystery.

But for all practical purposes, and we are all about being practical, these various other bodies and planes of existence have very limited impact on life in the physical realm.

They do exist, as do all the other realities, such as past lives, future lives, parallel lives etc; but just knowing and recognising that they are there is quite enough.

They don't really impact our normal day-to-day lives in any concrete way so they are, consequently, and just for the moment, fairly unimportant.

Many 'New Age' people, of course, will totally disagree.

They'll say developing these bodies along with the different abilities available within them is most important. They'll say to neglect these parts of yourself and not to explore these other realms is to limit your true potential.

And we have no problem with this way of thinking, if it is what you truly believe.

But we would just ask you to consider this...

Be physical in this physical universe

We've chosen to be physical in a physical universe.

The important words here are chosen and physical. We had the choice to be non-physical but we decided against it, we wanted to experience being All That Is through physical means.

Why therefore, having made this choice, should we then be trying to develop and experience these non-physical parts of ourselves?

To us it just seems to be an unnecessary waste of energy to be focusing on something we have chosen, in the first place, not to be.

The same could be said of these people who spend their whole lives in continual meditation in some cave up a mountain in Tibet or somewhere.

Why are they doing it?

It would seem, to us, that these people - far from displaying profound spiritual understanding — are missing the point completely.

You have come to a physical universe to be physical, so BE physical.

Don't worry about all these other bodies and other planes of existence for now. They are there, and they're already a part of you.

It can be no other way.

They will not disappear and your 'spirituality' will not suffer, even if you don't give them any energy at all. Far better, we think, to concentrate instead, on understanding physical life from a physical perspective.

It is, after all, the reason you came.

You see, there are too many people going around trying to be something they're not, out of a profound misunderstanding of who they are and why they're here.

They think spiritual 'growth' has to be about withdrawing from life and that only by dedicating oneself purely to meditation, chanting, ritual, and prayer will it be possible for spiritual understanding and enlightenment to manifest itself.

Just know that none of this is necessary.

What is the point of struggling and striving to be what you already are.

You already are fully enlightened for you are All That Is.

You just don't remember this fact yet, that's all.

Okay then. We hope by now you're beginning to realise (to make real) just how powerful you really are - and this power within you really is the divine power of All That Is...

Because it'll really help you understand your self-attunement.

So, it's about time we covered a little more about the subject of Reiki.

And please don't worry.

All the areas we've just spoken about will become clear, in the fullness of time, particularly when your own vibratory level begins to be raised back up again through your Reiki attunements.

So, what better place to start our visit back to Reiki than with:

The History of Reiki

If you already know about or don't want to know about this, please feel free to skip on to the next section.

We quite understand.

Okay then – if you're coming with us - let's get going...

There are presently two different versions of how Reiki came to be 're-discovered' doing the rounds.

There's the 'Western' version and the 'Eastern' version, and we'll look at the 'Western' version first.

It goes something like this.

Western version

In the mid 1800's, the Meiji period, Dr Mikao Usui was the dean of a small Christian university called Doshisha University in Kyoto Japan.

During one of his classes several students wanted to know whether he believed in the Bible.

Dr Usui replied that he did indeed believe.

The students then asked if he believed in Jesus' ability to heal the sick. Again Dr Usui replied he did. The students pressed his beliefs further.

They quoted Jesus' statement "You can do this too, and more", and asked when, if Dr Usui also accepted this as being true, they would be taught how to heal just like Jesus.

Now Dr Usui was a Japanese of very traditional values.

He was not able to pass these teachings on to his students and honour demanded that he resign.

He did so, immediately.

Dr Usui leaves Japan

He decided he would make it his life's mission to seek out the ability to heal as Jesus had done and went off in search of this knowledge.

He reasoned, as Jesus was a Christian, he'd find this knowledge in a Christian country and travelled to America.

On his arrival in America Dr Usui studied at the University of Chicago. But, despite spending seven years studying Christianity, philosophy, the scriptures and several other religions, he was unable to find the knowledge he sought.

He'd learned that Jesus was said to have travelled throughout India and Tibet and so decided that he too would follow in his footsteps.

Further studies in Buddhism

It was here that Dr Usui learned Sanskrit and studied the Indian and Tibetan Sutras. But still he was unable to find what he sought and so decided to travel back to Japan to further his studies in Buddhism, as he knew Buddha had also healed the sick.

Kyoto, at that time, had all the largest monasteries so naturally Dr Usui continued his search there.

He visited every monastery in turn, asking the monks whether they were able to heal as Buddha had done. The response from each monastery was always the same.

No.

They were aware that Buddha had healed the physical body and that it was written in the Sutras.

However it was their belief that healing the spirit was more important and because of this they didn't know how to heal the body.

Dr Usui was becoming more and more despondent but he didn't give up his search.

He continued on and came across a Zen monastery.

It was here that he met with great support for his search.

Even though the monks at this monastery were also concentrating on healing the spirit they believed the knowledge for healing the body would be made available to them through meditation.

And they invited Dr Usui to join them.

Nearing the end of his search

He spent three years there, searching the Sutras and meditating with the other monks, and eventually he discovered a formula for contacting a higher power able to bestow on the seeker abilities for healing the physical body.

This formula was, in itself, very simple, but it was going to need interpreting and testing to see if it worked.

Through meditation and discussion with the other monks, Dr Usui came to the realisation that enlightenment on how to use the formula would be given to him if he fasted and meditated for 21 days.

Mount Kurama

Near Kyoto was a very holy mountain called Mount Kurama, so it was the place Dr Usui travelled to. He climbed the mountain and found a beautiful spot, facing east, with water for drinking nearby.

To prevent himself from losing track of time he gathered together 21 stones with the intention of throwing away one stone at the dawn of each new day.

Ready for whatever experience that presented itself, Dr Usui began his vigil.

Dr Usui sees the light

For twenty days Dr Usui fasted, meditated, read the scriptures, chanted and prayed without anything out of the ordinary happening.

Then on the morning of the twenty-first day whilst looking out into the darkness of the pre-dawn he noticed what seemed to be a small flicker of light away in the distance.

As Dr Usui focussed on this light it began to travel towards him becoming brighter and brighter.

He became very afraid and was in two minds as to whether to stay or run away. Calming himself he remembered that this was the very reason he was there.

He stood up and determined that he would stay where he was and accept anything that happened, even if that meant his own death.

The light continued to get closer becoming much brighter as it did so.

Dr Usui was suddenly aware that the light was actually a consciousness and was seeking to communicate with him.

It said that this was the enlightenment to healing others that he'd been seeking. He was to understand however that the light would have to strike him in the third eye, and it was so powerful it might actually kill him.

The decision to allow this to happen was entirely up to Dr Usui, it had to be his own choice.

The light strikes

Dr Usui decided to allow the light to strike him.

The force of the blow knocked him unconscious and it was whilst he was in this trance like state that he saw beautiful bubbles of coloured lights rising up before his eyes.

Inside the bubbles were different symbols and as he studied them he became attuned to their energy.

When Dr Usui regained full consciousness he knew that what had transpired had been all that he had been looking for.

He felt tremendously energised and not at all weary.

Quickly he got his few possessions together, he wanted to get back to the monastery to share his experiences with the abbot.

The first miracle

Setting off at a great pace he stumbled, stubbing his toe quite badly in the process. The pain lanced through his body and he instinctively bent down and cupped the damaged toe in his hands. Immediately the pain began to subside and a few minutes later both the pain and the bleeding had stopped completely.

Dr Usui was thrilled. It was like a miracle.

There was something very different about his hands now.

They seemed to have emanated a tremendous heat whilst he was holding his toe.

Quickly he got back to his feet and hurried off down the mountain in the direction of the monastery.

At the foot of the mountain he came across a typical Japanese snack bar that had been set up to feed weary travellers. Dr Usui stopped and, with great enthusiasm, ordered a full breakfast.

The proprietor warned Dr Usui to only have a light meal of rice gruel. He could see by Dr Usui's unkempt and unshaved condition that he had obviously been meditating and, therefore, fasting for some time.

He didn't want his first customer of the day getting indigestion.

Dr Usui, however, felt so good he ignored the concerns of the proprietor and ate heartily, finishing the complete meal with no ill effects whatsoever.

Another miracle!

Dr Usui heals his first patient

As Dr Usui was preparing to pay for the meal the proprietor's granddaughter came to clear away the dishes.

He noticed tears in her eyes and that the side of her face was very red and swollen.

She appeared to be in great pain.

On enquiring from the proprietor as to why this was, he learned that the young girl had been suffering severe toothache for many days.

He also learned that the proprietor was unable to afford either the time or the money to take his granddaughter to the dentist seventeen miles away in Kyoto.

Overwhelmed with compassion

Dr Usui was overwhelmed with compassion and asked for permission to attempt to heal her.

The girl gladly accepted this offer of help and allowed Dr Usui to gently cup her face in his hands. Within seconds the discomfort began to subside and minutes later the pain and the swelling had completely disappeared.

A third miracle!

With the profuse thanks of the proprietor and the girl ringing in his ears Dr Usui set off on the rest of his journey back to the monastery.

On arrival he learned that the abbot had been laid up in bed with an acute attack of arthritis.

Wasting no time he went to his old friend and whilst recounting his experiences on the mountain gently rested his hands on the abbot's body. Again within moments the discomfort began to subside and minutes later had disappeared altogether. The abbot was astonished at this demonstration of healing and as the two friends talked into the night it was decided that the best thing to do next would be to go out into the city to heal the sick.

Dr Usui chose to go out and take up residence in the Beggars Kingdom.

He spent the next seven years working in this poor part of Kyoto, helping as many people as he could.

Many remarkable healings took place and Dr Usui was content with his life until he came across a beggar that he had healed many years before.

Dr Usui questioned this man as to why he had returned once more to the life of a beggar, and was extremely dismayed at the response.

It turned out that the beggar had been, initially, very happy at having been healed. He'd gone back into the main part of the city and had even found himself a good job. For a while he'd prospered but the responsibility of looking after himself became too much for him.

It was much easier living the life of a beggar.

Unfortunately this was not an isolated case. Dr Usui discovered more and more people who had returned to begging after having been healed, and it greatly saddened him.

Perhaps, he thought, the Buddhist monks were right. Perhaps it was more important to heal the spirit than the body.

Reiki should not be given for free

Dr Usui went into meditation to seek the answers on how he could have got it so wrong.

He discovered his biggest mistake was in healing the bodies of the beggars without teaching them the value of responsibility. He also realised that because he had been giving away the healing for free, none of the beggars had apportioned any value to this help.

Dr Usui had unwittingly strengthened their belief in begging as being the only way of getting what they wanted.

With this realisation he immediately closed his healing practice and left the Beggars Quarter.

It was also during this period that Dr Usui developed his Five Principles of Reiki, and became aware that the symbols he had been shown on Mount Kurama were to be used for initiating others into this healing system he now called Reiki.

For his remaining years Dr Usui travelled the length and breadth of Japan spreading his Reiki healing.

On his death in 1926 he had initiated 16 people as Reiki Masters and had charged one of his most dedicated students, Dr Chujiro Hayashi, with the responsibility of preserving and continuing the Reiki teachings.

1. Just for today, I will let go of anger.
2. Just for today, I will let go of worry.
3. Today, I will count my many blessings.
4. Today, I will do my work honestly.
5. Today, I will be kind to every living creature.

The Five Principles of Reiki

Dr Chujiro Hayashi

A retired naval officer, a commander in the Imperial Navy of Japan, Dr Hayashi was forty-seven when he was initiated as a Reiki Master.

He had spent many years following Dr Usui on his travels around Japan and had become a very capable and dedicated healer in his own right. It came as no surprise, therefore, that Dr Usui, much impressed with this competent leader of men, rewarded him by passing to him the title of Reiki Grand Master prior to his death.

Dr Hayashi went on to open the first Reiki clinic in Tokyo and it was here whilst using a combination of observation and clinical record keeping that he developed the twelve basic hand positions in use today.

For more on The 12 Hand Positions of Reiki, please go here:

http://www.chikara-reiki-do.com/reiki-hand-positions/

He also refined the attunement process by dividing it into three separate levels called degrees.

It's not known how many people Dr Hayashi trained in Reiki but it is known that, being a renowned psychic, Dr Hayashi foresaw the coming of the Second

World War and decided to pass on Reiki to two women.

This he did in the knowledge that many of the men he had trained would be killed in the fighting and he wanted to ensure that Reiki survived.

The two women he trained were his wife and Mrs Hawayo Takata.

Chapter 13: The Reiki Division

Dr. Mikao Usui taught three main levels or degrees of Reiki, which must be kept intact in their essence. All levels are activated with initiations that, as we saw, are also called chakras activations. The student who receives the first level, according to their convenience, can stop there or learn other levels and deepen the studies.

Several teachers, at present, divide the third level of Reiki into two phases (the inner teacher and the outer teacher) to understand that the student, to apply the technique of mastery in his personal life, must not necessarily undergo prolonged training (approximately seven months). It is also expensive for a teacher. Therefore, the so-called level 3-A is taught in quick seminars and the so-called "teacher" as level 3-B. Reiki seminars are presented in classroom periods ranging from eight to eighteen hours, according to the number of students and the teacher's teaching ability.

Some teachers recommend a time not less than three months between one level and the next. Other teachers, such as the American teacher Lori George, who lives in Northpend, USA, prefer intensive Reiki. All original initiations are performed in a single activation. All the resources of Reiki are placed at the disposal of the student in a single initiation, and it is at the discretion of the initiate how quickly he will advance. It is logical that Reiki energy is not going to harm him, but the twenty-one-day energy cleaning process can, in certain cases, present difficulties for the student, in addition to not being able to have enough time to understand the deep meaning of each level.

Level I or Physical (The Awakening)

The first level is also known as physical because the transmission of Reiki energy occurs by contact through the hands of the therapist on the patient.

Conforrne already said that anyone could receive the first level of Reiki, not having a special prerequisite: the knowledge transmitted is simple and scarce. What is basically taught are the positions of the hands. That's why no special prior knowledge is necessary to learn the Reiki technique.

Tuned people are trained to channel the cosmic vital energy through their hands, simply by placing them on those who must be harmonized, including themselves, animals, and plants. It is not necessary to direct the mind, concentrate, say prayers, believe or desire a cure. Reiki does not need our approval to act. The first level of Reiki is complete in itself. The channels will remain open for the rest of the Reikian's life, even though the initiate does not use the energy for prolonged periods. There is no need to receive another tuning on the same level. Throughout the world, it is common for the initiate to participate, free of charge, in seminars of the same level as other teachers.

At level I, the time of a complete treatment in oneself or in another person takes 60 to 90 minutes. After the four phases of initiation that lead to level I, the exchange of Reiki energy between

Reikians is recommended for four consecutive days, with the aim of clearing the energy channels opened during the performances. But that is not a rule. This exchange will provide more security to the practitioner who will also experience the experience as a Reiki recipient.

It is convenient to start with yourself daily and then give treatment to family and friends. This practice will not have the effect of improving the quality of the energy that flows from your hands, but it will enrich your baggage of knowledge, in relation to times and positions that aim to reach the most important energy centers (chakras), meridians and organs, in search of a complete harmonization.

In the first seminar, the Reikian will also learn the history of Reiki. In the first level seminars, we almost always observe the same phenomenon of participants' behavior. They start the seminar with a rather skeptical attitude; they do not talk to each other, and they do not externalize their feelings. It is as if they were isolated from the world. After tuning, they begin to talk, smile, and play. In the end, they behave as if they were former friends.

Level II or Mental (the Transformation)

This is also known as the mental level because the initiate will work with mental and emotional problems. The second level seminar takes place in a period similar to that of the first, from eight to eighteen hours. On that occasion, an initiation is made to three sacred Reiki symbols, which are taught and tuned into the hands of the participant. The different types of treatments depend on the combination of these three symbols.

We make the second level when we feel a need for greater growth and greater knowledge in relation to energy. The tuning process provides a jump in the vibratory level, at least twice as high as that experienced in level I. The symbols taught can also be used to send energy at a distance, to the past, and to the future.

Level II places great emphasis on the adjustment of the subtle body (mental/emotional) and not of the physical body, which is the focal point at the level I, and the student goes through a cleaning period of twenty-one days again.

Level II is not an improvement of the first since each one is a complete and perfect module that closes in itself. It should not be implied that the student of the second level is a better channel than that of the first, or that the personal treatment of the second is superior. In general, when we reach the second level, we value the first one even more.

The student who receives the initiation of the second level needs much less time than before, more or less, 15 to 20 minutes. It is worth noting that, with the symbols, healing also occurs on a physical level, in great intensity, due to the enhanced vibrations involved in the process. On the second level, we have to re-base the current way of explaining the concepts of time and space (distance) because when we work with symbols, energy acts in another dimension, where the "continuum" of time and space occurs.

Level III-A or Awareness (Completion)

It is also known as inner teacher degree or awareness. The student learns the mastery symbol and will be able to realize their wishes and dreams. This initiation does not yet qualify the student to teach Reiki: its use is limited to personal use.

Good teachers pay great attention to the time elapsed between that and the previous level so that there is a deep and conscious maturation, also avoiding an accumulation of crises from the cleaning process that follows the initiation, thus remaining lighter. This period, between levels II and III, can vary from four to twelve months. The third level requires extreme care since the volume of energy involved in the healing process is very large, and it is important to try to maintain a healthy diet and do personal development exercises.

At that level, we receive a sacred symbol that serves to amplify and intensify the effects of the symbols received in the second level, enabling the student to harmonize and heal a large number of people, a crowd, states, and even countries. We can be agents of planetary regeneration. The third level leads the student to find their most real truth to touch their own karma, the stage of conscious and constant learner.

Level III-B or Mastership

Level III-B is that of Reiki teacher, also called spiritual or teacher. The person who is tuned in as a Reiki teacher receives the knowledge of how to start new Reikians. That initiation does not force anyone to teach, and, in this way, more and more people decide to make such a choice within a perspective of inner growth. That training requires approximately seven months of training.

It is essential for the new teacher to consider and respect the work done by all the teachers that preceded him. The Reiki master is a person trained to initiate other people and cannot and should not be taken as an example, from a moral, ethical, or spiritual point of view. At the time of activation, all Reiki masters are equal. The variation occurs in the didactic ability to transmit the theoretical knowledge that is necessary.

Having received the teaching initiation does not guarantee that the new teacher is personally oriented. He must learn not to express opinions in seminars regarding the personal political, philosophical, religious, ideological, or spiritual beliefs of the students since Reiki harmonizes perfectly with all of them, making them stronger and clear in some cases. Students are absolutely free and without any degree of dependence in relation to the teacher or the institution to which they may belong.

The teacher, upon receiving the initiation to the master, assumes the commitment to transmit Reiki in the way it has been carried out from rediscovery. It is common to give assistance to all practitioners, regardless of the teacher with whom they have studied.

Chapter 14: Other Self-Healing Techniques

What Is Healing Touch?
Unlike Reiki, before you can exercise it, Healing Touch does not involve a tuning. It is a modality that Janet Mentgen, R.N. has created. And it was for those in the medical sector initially. It's accessible to all, though. It's a modality of energy, like Reiki. Several concentrations exist. 15 hours or more is basis for Level I training that enables individuals of different backgrounds to join, recognize their prior learning and further develop energy-based treatment ideas and abilities. There is also a need for powerful personal growth engagement and an understanding of holistic health values. Between these concentrations, there is no necessary waiting period, and they can teach each weekend, it is vital to have a knowledge of the 12 meridians and the chakras in

healing touch, also known as therapeutic touch, and to learn
hands-on therapeutic abilities in opening blocked energies. It needs mild practitioner-to-receiver use of hands. For particular circumstances such as back issues, Healing Touch has more methods available. Healing Touch is a way to change the energy system of the body in order to impact self-healing.

What Is Reiki?

Reiki channels the universal life energy is known as qi to boost mental, body, and spirit integration to improve the natural healing system. A Buddist Monk named Mikao Usui developed it in 1922. He taught the exercise to over 2,000 students before his death. Reiki can generally be trained in a weekend like Healing Touch. While many organizations give practitioners certificates, these courses are not formally regulated.

Before they can exercise on others, Reiki practitioners must be aligned. If the qi of the practitioner is blocked, their healing abilities will be hindered. The strokes in

Reiki are comparable to those observed in Healing Touch but are performed near the body, not directly on the body. This could create Reiki for those who dislike being touched a more comfortable exercise.

The Difference Between Healing Touch and Reiki

Healing Touch and Reiki are comparable alternative medicines, but the two differ significantly. Both are regarded as a form of alternative medicine known as energy medicine. Blocked energies can be published in both Healing Touch and Reiki that can assist promote the healing of many fundamental illnesses and illnesses. The concept behind both is that the physician can

channel the patient's life energy to encourage the process of healing to start. Many think these procedures encourage the body to heal itself without any additional medical intervention.

Although there are no clinical findings to demonstrate these allegations, the results of Reiki and Healing Touch swear by many patients.

Incorporating Reiki Healing into Your Yoga Practice

Guess what's missing from your yoga practice? (Hint: Reiki)

You've got a dozen yoga mats, a few stylish yoga outfits, and a few props. Your previous courses of yoga, books, and videos make sure you have down pat your poses and sequences. But as you advanced along your yoga trip, you may have begun to feel that something was missing from your exercise at home, something that could bring you to a greater, more enlightened plane.

That something you're lacking maybe that thing called Reiki.

Reiki Healing and Life Force Energy

Reiki is an ancient Japanese healing method that includes transferring "life force energy" or prana to particular areas of the body by laying hands on it. Reiki masters have effectively unlocked their prana free flow and can transfer Reiki's capacity to learners through a method known as "attunement." Once your own prana is unlocked and you have the capacity to use Reiki, you can use it on others or yourself, concentrating the energy of life force on particular areas of the body that can assist cure wounds and encourage excellent general health and wellbeing.

There are several including Yoga, Tai chi, Ayurveda, Acupuncture, Reflexology, Qi Do, Qi Gong, therapeutic touch, Bioresonance, and acupressure. What you are looking for may determine which of these (or others) you choose to techniques! Reiki is common because learning and mastering are simple. Qi Gong, Qi Do, and other comparable arts are more difficult because you need to construct your private energy to work with others.

Yoga For Unity and Balance

The term 'yoga' means 'joughing' or 'uniting.' This is much more than just a workout, despite the popular misconception that yoga is a type of exercise. This ancient discipline originating in India, enables one to unite body and mind at a fundamental stage. Yoga tries to unite the person with the universal at a deeper level. Yoga teaches you how to relax and release tension, and how to reinforce and stretch stiff muscles. It also helps balance and integrates mind, body, and spirit increases power flow and boosts the natural healing procedures of the body itself. Yoga approaches wellness in a holistic way as a strong form of mind-body medicine, acknowledging that physical ailments also have mental and spiritual elements. Yoga is an extensive self-development and transformation scheme at its core.

☐ Stress relief. Scientific studies have found that yoga lowers blood pressure and decreases amount of stress hormones secreted.

☐ Higher immunity. Yoga increases the ability of the body to fight against infections by enhancing flow of the lymphatic system.

☐ Flexibility and balance. With yoga, tight muscles release to enable increase in motion. So long as it is continuous, body awareness deepens enabling improvement in posture.

☐ Strength. Yoga is a powerful exercise that builds strength in every part of the body, including core muscles. This exercise helps prevent both muscular and skeletal problems, strengthening your body, build your inner strength, discipline, and self-confidence.

☐ Enhanced mood. Yoga enhances the release of endorphins by balancing the central and endocrine nervous system. During the process, you stop dwelling on life's stress as your mind relaxes, as said by Chopra in Yoga Can Heal Your Life, 2019.

Yoga and Life Force Energy

Yoga also has a strong focus on the flow of prana throughout the body, with the goal of unlocking and releasing the energy of your life force by moving into and holding different poses. Each time you hold a pose successfully while breathing profoundly, the blockages that stop your prana flow are efficiently dissolved. Different poses can unlock your prana in different ways. For example, forward bends can unblock prana to soothe, calm and ground you, while backbends prompt prana to revitalize you. Ironically, when it comes to dealing with the ailments of contemporary life— which can be exacerbated by severe pressure and a relentlessly fast-paced life— thousand-year-old techniques of healing could be some of the finest remedies.

The explosive popularity of meditation and yoga in the West— the advantages of physical and mental health are backed by a wide range of scientific research Put old techniques of healing on the map. Besides the more common practices of mindfulness, there are many more time-consuming (but still science-supported) self-healing techniques that you may not have heard of can work wonders to boost your health and well-being. As said by the early Greek physician, Hippocrates, "The natural healing power within each of us is the biggest strength to get well." Here are five old methods of self-healing that may be worth attempting.

Tai Chi

Like yoga, with a host of scientifically supported physical and mental health advantages, this calming, low-impact practice goes along. Originally, Tai Chi was created as a form of Chinese martial art and moving meditation, focusing on attention, breath, and motion. The practice is believed to unlock the Chinese notion of qi, the flowing energy force through the body, and to encourage adequate flow. Studies have discovered that Tai Chi can help enhance the quality of treatment of life for women with breast cancer when used to complement traditional therapy,

retain bone density, decrease pain in knee patients with serious osteoarthritis, encourage heart health, decrease high blood pressure, and more. According to Peter M. Wayne the director of the Tai Chi, there is currently a research for tai chi as an adjunct for standard medical treatment for rehabilitations of age associated conditions.

Ayurveda

As meditation and yoga's popularity has increased in the U.S., so has interest in Ayurveda, the 5,000-plus-year-old Indian "life science" that deals with healing through food, lifestyle, and herbal supplements. The theory is that Ayurveda can help cure imbalances in the doshas of the body— the three fundamental kinds of power— which include pitta (the principle of conversion; the element of fire), vata (the energy of movement; the element of air), and Kapha (the principle of development; the element of life). Ayurvedic practitioners think that each individual has some vata, pitta, and Kapha in them, but that one or two are typically dominant, the University of Maryland Medical Center describes: "Many things can disturb the equilibrium of energy, such as stress, unhealthy diet, climate, and strained family relationships. Although Ayurveda is understood in the West, a preliminary study has examined the efficacy of Ayurvedic programs in treating depression, anxiety, hypertension, Alzheimer's and other medical conditions.

Ayurvedic medicine should be used under a qualified practitioner's guidance, some may be dangerous, especially if misused.

Acupuncture

Some may find acupuncture unattractive — after all, it involves pricking lots of small needles into your skin — but a study has shown that ancient Chinese medicinal practice can actually function. Like Tai Chi, acupuncture attempts to balance the flow of qi throughout the body by inserting needles throughout the body into certain pathways or meridians. According to the Mayo Clinic, Western professionals tend to see the practice as a manner to boost blood flow by stimulating the nerves, muscles, and connective tissue in different areas of the body.

Research has demonstrated that acupuncture can be useful in treating headaches, high blood pressure, depression, back pain, nausea, rheumatoid arthritis, and other diseases.

As the New York Times made in 2010, Doctors are accepting acupuncture and are sending patients for boost in blood flow among others.

Reiki

The strength of contact can cure a range of distinct physical ailments and alleviate stress, as said by the practitioners. The physician positions his or her hands over different areas of the patient's body in a Reiki session, with the aim of guiding and stimulating the flow of "life force energy." As the International Center for Reiki Healing states, "Reiki treats the whole individual including body, emotions, mind, and spirit creating many useful impacts that include relaxation and feelings of peace, safety, and well-being." While there is restricted (and conflicting) research on the advantages of Reiki at this stage, some studies have suggested that Reiki may

be useful in decreasing anxiety, stress, and pain, enhancing symptoms of fatigue and depression, and boosting well-being. The method has begun to become more accepted in the West and is increasingly being used in U.S. hospitals, along with more standard care, as well as holistic health care facilities as part of a general mental care plan.

Reflexology

Reflexology is believed to enhance health by applying stress to particular areas of the hands, legs, and ears using "body mapping," a system that connects these pressure points with different organs and structures throughout the body.

Some studies have found reflexology to be useful in decreasing pain, anxiety, and depression, as well as encouraging relaxation and stress relief, the Mayo Clinic stated, but it has not yet been endorsed by allegations that reflexology can treat diseases such as asthma and diabetes.

Huffpost, (December 7, 2017)

Qi Gong

Qi gong (pronounced: chee-gun), which The fundamental exercise scheme in Chinese medicine incorporates meditative and physically active components. Qigong exercises are intended to assist maintain your Jing, reinforce and balance the flow of Qi energy and help understand your Shen. It's dynamic exercises and meditations combine Yin and Yang aspects: The Yin is being it; while Yang is doing it. Yin qigong exercises are articulated through relaxed stretching, breathing and image processing.

Yang qigong exercises are more aerobically or dynamically articulated. They are especially efficient in promoting the immune system. Qigong is widely used in China for individuals with cancer. Through the Twelve Primary Channels and Eight Extra Channels, Qigong's physical and spiritual routines move Qi energy, balance it, smooth the flow, and strengthen it. Chinese medicine utilizes Qigong exercises to preserve health, deter disease, and extend longevity, as it is a strong instrument to preserve and restore harmony with the organs, essential substances, and channels. Qigong is also used for non-medical reasons, such as combat and enlightenment pursuits.

Several Other Types of energy healing techniques exist are as follows;

- Quantum Touch
- Restorative Touch
- Shamanic Healing
- Theta Healing
- Chakra balancing
- Energy-Focused Bodywork
- Magnetic healing

Quantum Touch

Quantum Touch focuses in particular on using the breath of the practitioner to intensify the therapy. Practitioners grow their own energy and bring the energy of the customer to this greater (healthier) stage.

Restorative Touch

Restorative Touch is a distinctive and strong type of energy work that operates on a resonance model to "promote health, healing, and spiritual evolution." Through rigorous certification and licensing procedures, practitioners are extremely educated and kept to high standards.

Shamanic Healing

Shamanic healers perform spiritual realm energy, calling for spiritual helpers like animals of authority or other spiritual forces. A variety of mental and physical diseases are treated with the shamanic role.

Theta Healing

This method is described by the Theta Healing as concentrating on thought and prayer, relying on God / Source to do the real healing. The patient comes into a theta brain wave state (profound meditation), as explained by the practitioner, asks God (or Source) for help and then witnesses the healing. Theta Healing argues that it is feasible to make instant physical and emotional changes.

Chakra balancing

Chakra, or "wheel" in Old Sanskrit, relates to the power of life (or prana, as stated above) moving within the human body. The seven primary chakras of the body channel optimum energy levels to each linked element of mind, body, and spirit when balanced. Unbalanced chakras— or power, however, that spins too fast or slowly— typically have adverse impacts on the health of the body. Starting with the Root chakra below the genitals and ending with the Crown chakra above the head's crown, this chakra graph sheds light on the significance of keeping the equilibrium in each of the seven chakras.

Energy-Focused Bodywork

As part of the power scheme, the body is often ignored. All is energy, though, and that implies the body is also energy. All bodywork (massage) affects your energy, but some types are deliberate about it.

Magnetic healing

These magnets are used to release emotions that are trapped which cause discomfort while increasing blood flow, enhancing flexibility, building muscle power, and relaxing and lengthening the muscles and soft tissues of the body. As described in The Emotion Code, after recognizing Trapped Emotions, magnetic healing is typically introduced when professionals pass three times

a magnet over the Governing Meridian in the patient's body. This exercise fills the body with magnetic energy when mixed with the practitioner's healing intentions, which helps free and transform the trapped emotional energy. Because the body works on biomagnetic energy values, muscle testing can be used to connect with the subconscious mind to define the forces and feelings that govern physical, mental, and emotional afflictions as narrated by Jagdish in 2017. So many others such as Healing Touch, Spiritual Healing, Intuitive Healing, Polarity Therapy, etc

Chapter 15: Understanding The Reiki Symbols

The Usui School and its variants make use of these symbols, but other schools do not. It's important to understand that the symbols are not holy or powerful in and of themselves. They act instead as a sort of meditative aid for practitioners who learn their use through formal training. There are many symbols used by different schools, but Usui taught four which are considered "traditional." These are:

Choku Rei—The Power Symbol

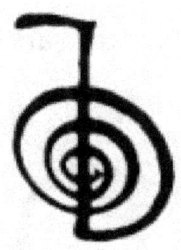

To reiki practitioners, this symbol means "put the universal power here." The horizontal bar on top symbolizes the source of reiki. The vertical line in the center represents the flow of reiki, while the spiral touches that line several times to represent how infinite that power is. Others say it represents the seven energy centers in the body (known as chakras) since it touches the central line seven times.

Some centers display this symbol, while others simply draw it in the air with their hands before a session. The belief is that not only does it dispel negative energy, it also boosts the practitioner's ability to tap into universal power and direct it as needed.

Sei He Ki—The Mental and Emotional Symbol

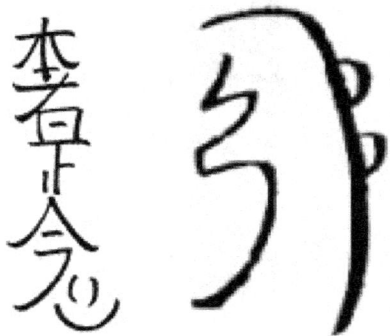

This means "god and (wo)man become one." The character on the left represents yang—the light, male, dominant, logical aspect; while the one on the right represents yin—the dark, female, submissive, intuitive aspect.

Reiki practitioners understand that not all ailments are purely of the body, but also of the mind and spirit. This symbol, therefore, helps to balance any mental and emotional imbalances which may be causing physical health problems.

Practitioners harness its power to treat mental and emotional problems that a patient might not even be aware of. It's therefore useful in helping those suffering from depression, stress, and trauma, as well as those with substance abuse issues. It's also used to boost memory, strengthen resolve (useful in weight loss), and improve creativity.

Hon Sha Ze Sho Nen—The Distance Healing Symbol

Many reiki practitioners believe it means "no past, no present, no future," though others claim it can also be understood as "the Buddha in me connects with the Buddha in you." Neither are correct.

The "hon sha ze sho nen" is not actually a symbol, but the Japanese pronunciation of an extremely clever combination of overlapping Chinese characters: 本者是正念. This translates into English as: "Correct thought/mindfulness is the essence of being."

This symbol is taught to advanced practitioners for distance healing. As such, "the Buddha in me connects with the Buddha in you," is a workable translation for the purposes of distance reiki. Since the practitioner cannot know what their absent patient might be going through, they invoke the power of this symbol to direct their healing thoughts to the person who needs their strength.

Dai Ko Myo—The Master Symbol

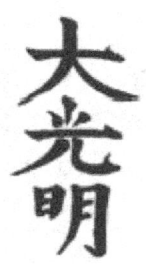

This literally translates into English as great(大) shining(明) light(光)," though practitioners understand it to mean the "great enlightenment." This symbol cleanses the body and invokes the healing power of compassion, insight, and clarity.

It's also associated with initiation, since advanced practitioners use it to bring about the attunement process among novices. This allows new practitioners to permanently access universal life force energy, both for themselves and for others.

Once acquired, this power can never be lost, though it should be developed and regularly harnessed through daily practice as described in Chapter 4.

Chapter 16: Testimonials And Stories

Perhaps you're wondering if all of the information you have read can be backed up by real-life experiences. The following stories and testimonials are experiences that real people have had. They are documented instances from Reiki recipients, practitioners, and even casual observers.

This first story is an instance in which a pet owner witnessed his girlfriend performing Reiki on their pet ferret when she was sick.

"I've never been a believer in Reiki or energy work. I still don't really understand it. When our ferret, Angel, got sick, she was lethargic, excessively drooling, and her eyes were glazed over. It was late at night and we were considering rushing to the emergency vet. For over a half-hour we sat on the couch with Angel and watched her suffer.

I started to play video games to keep myself calm and that is when my girlfriend started doing Reiki on our ferret. I didn't know what she was doing at first, but then I saw her draw some symbols over Angel and assumed it was Reiki. In just minutes, Angel stopped drooling and started to stretch. After only five minutes, Angel was back to her wiggly, energetic self!

I can only describe what I saw as miraculous.

Over the next few months, there were more instances where Angel would become lethargic, start to drool and become weak, and have glazed eyes. Whether she was in that state for ten minutes or over an hour, just five minutes of Reiki from my girlfriend would completely return Angel to her normal energy levels!

It was truly incredible and gave us several more months with our beloved Angel."

Kristopher

Reiki is a powerful healing modality for both people and animals. A man who has no previous interest or belief in Reiki witnesses its healing power and then describes it as miraculous. Even without understanding how it works or what happened, he could visibly see the change it made in his pet when she was sick.

The next story we come to is from a Reiki Master who runs a private bodywork practice and sees clients for Massage, Reiki, and Shamanic work. It is the story of an experience she had with a specific client.

"Many of my massage clients know that I also offer Reiki sessions and Shamanic Healing sessions. One of my regular clients has been coming to see me for weekly 2-hour massages for over a year. He has asked me about Reiki on several occasions, so finally, when he had the time, he decided to get a Reiki session and try it out.

After the session, we discussed what he had felt or experienced. He said he didn't experience much, but he did see a lot of shades of purple during the session. As we wrapped up our day, I told him that some people will feel the effects of Reiki immediately while other people won't notice anything until later. I also said that Reiki isn't for everyone and some people try it out and decide that they don't want to continue with treatments for whatever reason.

He told me that he thinks that he is the kind of person who doesn't think he will get any benefit out of Reiki. I was disappointed, but I didn't push the matter.

When this client came to see me for his weekly massage a few days later, he was very excited to tell me about his follow up experience after our Reiki session. He told me that when he went home, he felt more energized than he had in a long time! He said that he was able to get so many projects around the house done that the felt like there wasn't enough time in the day to keep working. He never felt worn out or tired.

Then, later in his workweek, there were two days where changes were made to his workload and schedule that normally would have caused him anger and stress. He said that rather than getting mad, he was able to just go with the flow and keep a positive mindset.

My client attributed both of these experiences to the Reiki session. He still comes to see me for 2-hour massages once a week, but now, he will often get combo sessions of both Reiki and massage.

To this day, I haven't had a client who has received a Reiki session and then not felt any benefit or been interested in getting another one."

Isabella

Since Reiki is subtle energy, sometimes, it can take time for the effects to be apparent. Educating your clients, as this Reiki Master did, is a good way to ensure that they know what to expect before and after a session.

This client didn't feel anything related to the Reiki session on the table but was aware enough to notice changes in his everyday life after the fact. Thus he could report back to his practitioner that he had experienced the benefit of Reiki and wanted to keep getting treatments.

The next story comes from a woman who had never heard of Reiki, but when her sister became a Reiki practitioner, she wanted to try it out and see what it was all about. She had gotten massages and spa treatments before, but she had never received energy work.

"I asked my sister to give me a Reiki session because I had never heard of it before but I figured I could try it out. I wanted to be supportive of what my sister was doing. I told her that I had been feeling very stressed about work and that I wanted to lose weight.

As soon as my sister started the session and put her hands on my head, I immediately felt like my entire brain was opening up. It was a very strange sensation. I just kind of let myself relax into the feeling because I was instantly relaxed by the work. All my stress just drained right away!

As my sister continued working, I realized that I had absolutely no awareness of my feet. Whatever normally connected my brain to the knowledge that my feet existed was just gone! It felt like they weren't there at all. It was strange, but not unsettling. Then when she got to my lower abdomen she drew a couple symbols on my body.

After the session, I told her how I had felt and she explained to me what to expect and how I might experience vivid dreams. She also cautioned me to drink plenty of water.

I returned home with my husband a few days later and resumed my normal life. I hadn't given much thought to my Reiki session until my husband pointed out that I hadn't been eating as big of portions at mealtimes. So I checked my weight and in only a week, I had lost around seven pounds! I hadn't even been consciously trying.

Now, I don't know if that was a subconscious placebo effect, but it worked. Whatever it was really worked. I hadn't even thought to keep track of my experiences until my husband made a comment. He hadn't even known I wanted to lose weight as one of the goals of my Reiki session. It wasn't like he was looking for weight-related results afterward.

I encouraged my sister to keep going with her Reiki practice because honestly, she made me a believer in the concept of energy work and I think she has a great gift to offer other people as well."

Olivia

Another story in which someone who doesn't have previous experience with energy work, and who might be a little skeptical, but had a transformative experience on the table. This woman's experience during the session was much more profound, and then she continued to receive benefits after the fact. Even when she hadn't been keenly focused on her session, another outside observer was the first to notice a change.

The following story is another story about an animal who was receiving Reiki. The story comes from the pet's owner who was present at every treatment session.

"My baby boy was diagnosed with thyroid cancer. My husband and I decided that we wanted to go with a holistic approach to treating him. We didn't want him to go through painful treatments or be in and out of veterinary hospitals for months at a time. So, a friend of ours got us in touch with a local Reiki practitioner who worked on animals.

Not only did our Reiki practitioner come to meet us and our dog first for a free consultation, but every session, she came right to our house. The free consultation allowed us to determine if she would be a good match to work with our dog, and she was! Then having her come to our home meant our boy could be comfortable and relaxed during his sessions.

We started getting biweekly treatments for our dog. He was on a lot of other supplements and holistic medications for treatment. It was comforting to know that the Reiki energy wouldn't interfere with his other treatments.

Right away, we noticed differences in our dog. Whenever she started a Reiki session, he would come right up to her and want to be next to her. He would try to get in her lap or just roll over and want her to touch him all over. He was so happy when she started working. Then he would get up and go lie down under his favorite table and completely pass out.

Our other dog, a thirteen-year-old lab who has never been that keen on strangers or cuddling, would then go up to our Reiki practitioner and start licking her hands and sit right up against her. It was so strange to see our lab being so affectionate and cuddly with someone she hardly knew! She must have sensed the energy.

Our Reiki practitioner began doing joint sessions on both our dogs. She would also use Reiki energy to clear our home and create a safe, relaxed space. My husband and I were present for all the sessions and we could really feel the difference in the atmosphere of our home. On the off weeks that we didn't have a session scheduled, we got in the habit of holding that same healing space for both our dogs at the same of day.

Over the months, we saw that our lovable baby boy would get so excited when our Reiki practitioner came over. He would run out to greet her and roll over and want her to touch him and pet him. It was great to see because we could tell that he was getting sicker. His energy levels weren't as high and his playfulness was waning, but seeing his reaction to her every time she came over was completely heartwarming.

We worked with a holistic vet as well who also told us that the tumor growth had slowed drastically since he had been receiving Reiki sessions.

My husband and I are so thankful that we found a Reiki practitioner who gave us several more good months with our baby."
Holly

While Reiki isn't a cure-all, it can still be powerful in treating terminal illnesses, or at least, reducing the symptoms, as this woman witnessed in her dog. Reiki is a complementary treatment that can be used alongside other treatments, therapies, medications, and supplements without any interference. This applies to both working with people and animals. Reiki has been known to be especially effective when treating cancer patients to relieve pain and the side effects of treatments.

In many cases with cancer treatments, the patients are lacking something as simple as physical touch. Having Reiki performed on them gives them a healing benefit and also provides them with physical contact. On a psychological level, that can be monumentally beneficial to patients being treated for invasive or terminal illnesses.

Our last story is from a woman who has traveled the world and had many different kinds of energy work and healing performed on her. She gets biweekly massages and biweekly Reiki sessions.

"I've experienced some incredible modalities over the years. When I found my Reiki practitioner though, everything for me changed. She brought my health and wellness to an entirely new level. I have received Reiki before and I've always been a little particular about who works on me, but when I found this practitioner, I knew right away that she was the perfect fit for me.

I have been struggling with a lot of health problems for years. Problems in my hips, low back, neck, and adrenal glands. When I started getting Reiki, the pain immediately began to release. Unfortunately, the relief would only last for a few days, so I balanced Reiki and massage. But every time I went in for a Reiki session, I would learn something new.

I had also been dealing with major changes in my personal life. I wasn't quite sure where I wanted to go or how I was going to move forward. Not only was I looking for relief from physical pain, but I was also needing direction and guidance on a more personal level.

The biggest struggle I was having was in deciding whether or not I wanted to change or leave a job that I'd had for years. It was no longer fulfilling and I felt like it was sucking the life out of me.

The practitioner I found was not only a skilled healer but would talk to me about everything she found during a session and anything she saw or felt. We would discuss in length the things she saw as well as the things that I would see. My mind would really travel when she worked on me.

It only took a couple of sessions with her for me to find the clarity I needed to change the course of my own life. The anxiety I had been feeling about leaving my job vanished and I knew it was the right course of action. I was finally able to move on with my own life and my own passions. I never would have had that without getting Reiki sessions.

After one session, my practitioner told me that she discovered a strong energy sensation in my C4 and C5 vertebrae. I had been experiencing worsening neck pain for a few weeks. With that information, I went to my doctor and they determined that I had begun developing arthritis in my C4 and C5 vertebrae. My whole neck had been hurting, but having my practitioner narrow down the source of the pain is what led me to seek out medical advice and now I have additional options for relieving my neck pains.

During my Reiki sessions, I began to notice that my breathing would change. Not only would I become more relaxed, but the pattern of my breathing would change. I mentioned this to my practitioner and she was able to keep a better eye on it. After a few more sessions, we talked about the changes in breathing.

Through our discussion and what I knew of my own family medical history, I thought it best to get tested for sleep apnea. It turned out I did have the preliminary development of sleep apnea. I was able to get on top of that development thankfully. Without Reiki, I wouldn't have been made aware of that odd change in my breathing and the sleep apnea could have gone along a lot longer without being addressed.

Additionally, as I kept going through my Reiki sessions, I was able to confront a lot of emotional baggage that I had been holding on to in regards to my own family. It was such a help to me physically and emotionally. I also made huge strides in my own medical treatments for a healthier lifestyle."

Deb

Coming from a recipient that received long term, regular Reiki treatments really outlines how beneficial it can be on multiple levels of healing and improving lifestyle.

Chapter 17: Mental, Emotional, And Spiritual Healing

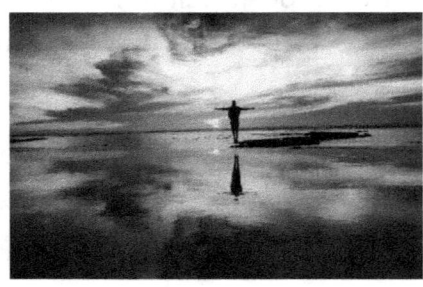

Sometimes ailments of the mind, emotional body, and spirit can be more debilitating than physical ailments. There are a few reasons for this. The first reason is that when the mind, emotions, and spirit are impacted it is usually an invisible pain that can't be measured by doctors and tools and can't visibly be seen by anyone else.

Unfortunately, this can lead to stigmas and unfair accusations that the pain isn't real or that the sufferer is making it up for attention or any other reason. Being in the position where this is the perception that others have of you can only add to the turmoil and the disease that impacts your mind, emotions, and spirit.

Sometimes these ailments can stem from a physical trauma, like physical abuse, but the lasting effects are mental, emotional, or spiritual. The physical body is just one layer in what makes a person. The western medical field has a strong focus on the physical body. This isn't necessarily a bad thing; however, it leaves the rest of the layers unnoticed and treats them as unimportant.

As more awareness about the different layers of people i.e. the emotional body and spiritual body, begins to grow and spread, disciplines like Reiki are becoming more popular and renowned. This is because therapies like Reiki have been used as a holistic healing method for centuries and Reiki does address all the different layers that can be impacted by imbalance and dis-ease.

When it comes to self-healing and personal power, having Reiki in your pocket as a tool that can be used is going to change the world for you. You'll have the ability make personal changes and shifts that may have seemed out of reach before. More than that, you'll have the ability to help yourself, even if no one else understands your suffering or thinks your suffering is real.

The truth is, everyone suffers, that is how change happens. Everyone experiences negativity, that is how they grow. With Reiki, you have the opportunity to help yourself and help others change and grow.

Some common ailments of the mind, emotional body, and spirit include:

Depression

Anxiety disorders

Eating disorders

Grief

Anger Management

Control issues

OCD (Obsessive Compulsive Disorder)

While the severity of these ailments can vary greatly, anyone who has struggled with these ailments knows that the degree doesn't matter when you are trapped in the pattern that your mind creates around these symptoms.

Depression

Depression is classified as a lack of dopamine and serotonin production in the brain. It is a chemical imbalance that leads to feelings of sadness, dread, fear, paranoia, feeling stuck, having a lack of self-worth, lack of self-love, having low energy and no motivation.

Some cases of depression are so severe that people won't get out of bed for days, or their appetite vanishes and if no one reminds them to eat they become very malnourished. Depression can be debilitating and contribute to anxiety and paranoia preventing people from being able to leave their homes.

In some cases, being severely depressed leads to self-harming tendencies and suicide. The common treatment for depression is medication and psychotherapy. Depression can be a result of trauma, abuse, or genetics. Sometimes there is no discernable reason.

Thankfully, awareness of mental health conditions like depression is growing. However, many people are still looking to alternative therapies such as Reiki to help with their depression. Medications can have side effects and most shouldn't be continued long term. Generally, people who are depressed are on more than one medication to stabilize themselves.

Reiki offers a noninvasive, nonpharmaceutical option to helping with depression symptoms. Reiki has been known to boost energy levels, increase motivation, and release energy related to traumas. Even if Reiki just opens the door to changes, like being able to take a walk every day, then the mind and body can begin healing the rest. It is the change from Reiki that allows you to take the next step in healing.

Anxiety Disorders

As with depression, awareness around anxiety disorders is becoming more prevalent and accepted. Anxiety disorders create an intense feeling of fear and worry within a person based on specific situations and circumstances. This fear and worry can result in trouble sleeping, hyperventilating, panic attacks, sweating, and physical illness. In more severe cases, anxiety can become a phobia.

Some phobias and anxieties are so severe that people can't leave their own homes. Many people with severe anxieties and phobias are treated through talk therapy and medications.

This is why Reiki is so beneficial, because it can be sent over time and space. If someone is too anxious to leave their homes, Reiki can be sent to them to help balance their dis-ease and relieve their anxieties. Additionally, if you have anxiety over social engagements, you can send Reiki to the time and place that you are engaging in a social activity. When you get there, the Reiki energy will be waiting for you to help ease your symptoms.

Grief

Grief is a deep-rooted sadness that stems from trauma, usually a loss of some kind. While it isn't the same as depression and it is more debilitating than regular sadness, grief can still disrupt everyday life.

When someone loses a loved one, family member, child, or pet, grief can become all consuming and they might not be able to move on. Letting go and moving on is the hardest part!

Reiki energy healing is all about releasing unneeded and unwanted energies, releasing imbalances and restoring balance. This is what makes it so effective in treating emotional imbalances such as excessive grief.

A certain amount of grief is healthy when it comes to loss. Excessive grief becomes the inability to move on, and that is when Reiki can become an asset.

Anger Management

Anger issues stem from a place of feeling powerless and out of control. There are different degrees of anger issues, some are more explosive and can even become violent. Part of the presentation of anger issues comes from society imposing the idea that all anger is bad and shouldn't be expressed.

When it doesn't get expressed, anger gets stored and becomes more and more dangerous for the person bottling it up and for the people around them. Most of the time, anger management issues are treated with talk therapy, support groups, and sometimes medication like mood stabilizers.

Reiki has a calming effect on the mind, body, and spirit. It creates a deep feeling of relaxation and also releases stored and blocked energies. If anger is something you struggle with, Reiki can help release what is stored, and the five Reiki principles can help you to change the way your mind and body react to potential anger in sighting situations.

Control Issues

Control issues are another ailment that originates from a place of feeling out of control or a lack of power. Control issues can manifest in many ways. Some people with control issues become meticulous and have to control every fine detail of their personal lives. Other people with control issues project them outward and start to micromanage the people around them.

From an energetic standpoint, control issues arise from an energetic imbalance in the solar plexus chakra. Reiki can help by balancing the solar plexus chakra, but Reiki helps in other ways as well. Through Gassho meditations you can learn to release and let go of that need for control. Reiki also increases your personal power and personal vibration, this essentially removes the lack of power feeling that creates a control issue.

OCD (Obsessive Compulsive Disorder)

OCD is a more prominent, severe kind of control disorder. The degrees of OCD vary and can be quite disruptive to everyday life. There is some evidence to suggest that OCD is a disorder where the brain doesn't have proper communication between various lobes. Treatment for OCD can be talk therapy and medication.

Unlike other disorders, depending on how severe OCD manifests, rationalization and logic can't override the OCD compulsions. The compulsions that manifest are often so programmed into the mind, and are a direct response to the way the brain communicates with the body, they become as natural and unconscious as your knee kicking out during a reflex test at the doctor's office. If a compulsive behavior isn't acted on, it creates a severe amount of anxiety within the person.

Reiki can greatly help reduce the symptoms of OCD which often include anxiety, paranoia, and phobias. Reiki can help with imbalances in the brain that might lead to OCD tendencies and compulsions. It can also release the energies that might be contributing to the compulsions.

As you can see, Reiki has so many uses when it comes to treating physical, mental, emotional, and spiritual ailments. Sometimes having it as a complimentary therapy to relieve symptoms is the best option. Other times, using it as a main treatment option yields the best results. Reiki is holistic and noninvasive and can be used in conjunction with medical treatments.

Self-Reiki treatments are going to be the best way for you to implement Reiki as a self-healing technique. There are other ways to utilize Reiki though, especially when it comes to mental, emotional, and spiritual healing. Meditation is going to be greatly beneficial to mental, emotional, and spiritual health. Reiki can be used in conjunction with meditation to achieve these goals.

To include Reiki in meditation, you can start or end your meditation with Gassho. You can perform your self-Reiki treatment before or after your meditation, or you can perform a meditation that directly incorporates Reiki into the process.

When you meditate, you'll want to find a quiet, secluded place where you can be alone and undisturbed for the duration of the meditation. You can make this space as relaxing and comfortable as you want, but be wary of falling asleep. Guided meditations are a great way to learn how to meditate if you are new to meditation.

Included in this chapter is a meditation exercise that is going to help you connect with Reiki energy and help you connect to your mind and spirit. This meditation will provide you with healing energy for the mind, emotions, and the spirit.

Meditation Exercise

Find a quiet, relaxing place where you can be alone and undisturbed. Sit down comfortably and close your eyes. Ask that you be open to receiving Reiki energy.

Take a deep breath in through your nose and out through our mouth. Feel the Reiki energy flowing though you. Breathe in deeply through your nose to the count of four and out through your mouth to the count of eight. Breathe in through the nose to the count of four and out through your mouth to the count of eight.

Continue to breathe deeply in through your nose and out through your mouth. Bring your hands together in the prayer position, your fingers touching and your palms spaced apart slightly.

Hold your hands about four inches from your body and have the tips of your fingers pointing towards the sky, level with your brow or nose.

In your third eye chakra, visualize the tips of your middle fingers with a bead of light at the top. Continue to breathe deeply in through the nose to the count of four and out through the mouth to the count of eight.

Hold that bead of light in your third eye chakra.

When you are called to, open your eyes and focus your attention on you're the tips of your middle fingers. Continue to breathe deeply in through your nose and out through your mouth. Set your focus to the tips of your middle fingers and if your mind begins to wander, refocus by pressing your middle fingers together.

Continue to focus on your middle fingers with your eyes open, breathing deeply in through the nose and out through mouth.

Close your eyes again and lower your hands into your lap. Take a deep breath in through the nose to the count of four and out through the mouth to the count of eight. Feel the Reiki energy in your hands. Perhaps your palms will feel warm or they will tingle with energy.

Keeping your eyes closed, raise your dominant hand and place your fingers against your third eye chakra at your brow and feel the connection between Reiki and your third eye.

Take another deep breath in through the nose and out through the mouth, lowing your fingers to your heart chakra at your sternum. Root the Reiki energy into your heart chakra before bringing your dominant hand back to your lap.

Breathe deeply in through the nose to the count of four and out through the mouth to the count of eight.

Raising your dominant hand again to the third eye chakra at your brow, place your fingers against your brow and breath deeply in through the nose and out through the mouth. Now bring your dominant hand up to your crown chakra and lay your palm flat against the top of your head. Breath Reiki energy into your crown chakra and feel the connection there.

Take a deep breath in through the nose to the count of four and out through the mouth to the count of eight.

Bring your hand back to your heart chakra and root the Reiki energy into your heart center. Then release your hand back to your lap and continue to breathe deeply in through the nose and out through the mouth.

In your mind's eye, visualize your crown chakra opening up to the cosmic universe and Reiki energy. Breathe in through your nose, drawing energy down through your crown chakra. Breathe out through the mouth to the count of eight. Breathe in again through your crown chakra, drawing Reiki energy down your spine and into the third eye chakra, throat chakra, heart chakra, solar plexus chakra, sacral chakra, and root chakra.

Let the Reiki energy release with your exhale out the root chakra down towards your feet.

Breathe in deeply through the crown chakra, drawing Reiki from the universe, through the crown and down the spine to the third eye chakra, throat chakra, heat chakra, solar plexus chakra, sacral chakra, and root chakra.

Breathe out through the mouth, releasing Reiki energy out of the root chakra and out towards the feet.

Take a deep breath in through the nose to the count of four and out through the mouth to the count of eight. Start to come back to your physical body. Breathe in through the nose and out through the mouth, connecting back to your skin. Breathe in through the nose and out through the mouth.

When you have completed your meditation, perform a grounding exercise if necessary.

Conclusion

Reiki is all about connections – it connects you to the energy of the universe gifting you with a new and abundant source of energy through which you can charge yourself. Reiki's purpose is to further these connections for you in the physical world, by connecting you to a whole sect of people who practice Reiki, and if you become a Reiki practitioner, to clients who you can further this energy too.

Our lives can only be studied by us in the physical form, which is why we erode and ignore the spiritual and the mental just because we cannot see them. Reiki asks only a simple thing from you, and that's your belief. If you believe in its power, and follow its values of compassion, there is nothing in your life that you cannot heal.

Thank you for buying this book, and I hope that it was an enriching and enlightening experience for you.

www.ingramcontent.com/pod-product-compliance
Lightning Source LLC
Chambersburg PA
CBHW072001070526
44583CB00015B/1288